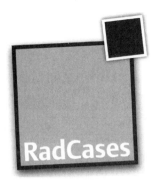

RadCases

# Gastrointestinal Imaging

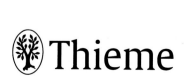

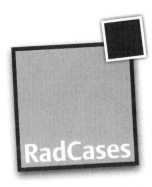

# Gastrointestinal Imaging

Edited by

**Jonathan Lorenz, MD**
Associate Professor of Radiology
Department of Radiology
The University of Chicago
Chicago, Illinois

Series Editors

**Jonathan Lorenz, MD**
Associate Professor of Radiology
Department of Radiology
The University of Chicago
Chicago, Illinois

**Hector Ferral, MD**
Professor of Radiology
Section Chief, Interventional Radiology
Rush University Medical Center, Chicago
Chicago, Illinois

Thieme
New York • Stuttgart

Thieme Medical Publishers, Inc.
333 Seventh Ave.
New York, NY 10001

Executive Editor: Timothy Hiscock
Editorial Assistant: Adriana di Giorgio
Editorial Director: Michael Wachinger
Production Editor: Katy Whipple, Maryland Composition
International Production Director: Andreas Schabert
Vice President, International Marketing and Sales: Cornelia Schulze
Chief Financial Officer: James W. Mitos
President: Brian D. Scanlan
Compositor: MPS Content Services
Printer: Sheridan Press

Library of Congress Cataloging-in-Publication Data

Gastrointestinal imaging / edited by Jonathan Lorenz.
    p. ; cm.—(RadCases)
  Includes bibliographical references.
  ISBN 978-1-60406-183-3
 1.  Gastrointestinal system—Imaging—Case studies.  I. Lorenz, Jonathan  II. Series: RadCases.
  [DNLM: 1.  Gastrointestinal Diseases—radiography—Case Reports. 2.  Diagnosis,
Differential—Case Reports. 3.  Gastrointestinal Tract-radiography—Case Reports.  WI 141]
  RC804.D52G37 2011
  616.3'307572—dc22
                                                                        2010040225

**Important note:** Medical knowledge is ever-changing. As new research and clinical experience broaden our
knowledge, changes in treatment and drug therapy may be required. The authors and editors of the material
herein have consulted sources believed to be reliable in their efforts to provide information that is complete
and in accord with the standards accepted at the time of publication. However, in view of the possibility of
human error by the authors, editors, or publisher of the work herein or changes in medical knowledge, nei-
ther the authors, editors, nor publisher, nor any other party who has been involved in the preparation of this
work, warrants that the information contained herein is in every respect accurate or complete, and they are
not responsible for any errors or omissions or for the results obtained from use of such information. Readers
are encouraged to confirm the information contained herein with other sources. For example, readers are
advised to check the product information sheet included in the package of each drug they plan to administer
to be certain that the information contained in this publication is accurate and that changes have not been
made in the recommended dose or in the contraindications for administration. This recommendation is of
particular importance in connection with new or infrequently used drugs.

Some of the product names, patents, and registered designs referred to in this book are in fact registered
trademarks or proprietary names even though specific reference to this fact is not always made in the text.
Therefore, the appearance of a name without designation as proprietary is not to be construed as a represen-
tation by the publisher that it is in the public domain.

Printed in the United States

978-1-60406-183-3

To my wife, Cynthia, and my son, Matthew, for their love and many sacrifices on my behalf.
*—Jonathan Lorenz*

# RadCases Series Preface

The ability to assimilate detailed information across the entire spectrum of radiology is the Holy Grail sought by those preparing for the American Board of Radiology examination. As enthusiastic partners in the Thieme RadCases Series who formerly took the examination, we understand the exhaustion and frustration shared by residents and the families of residents engaged in this quest. It has been our observation that despite ongoing efforts to improve Web-based interactive databases, residents still find themselves searching for material they can review while preparing for the radiology board examinations and remain frustrated by the fact that only a few printed guidebooks are available, which are limited in both format and image quality. Perhaps their greatest source of frustration is the inability to easily locate groups of cases across all subspecialties of radiology that are organized and tailored for their immediate study needs. Imagine being able to immediately access groups of high-quality cases to arrange study sessions, quickly extract and master information, and prepare for theme-based radiology conferences. Our goal in creating the RadCases Series was to combine the popularity and portability of printed books with the adaptability, exceptional quality, and interactive features of an electronic case-based format.

The intent of the printed book is to encourage repeated priming in the use of critical information by providing a portable group of exceptional core cases that the resident can master. The best way to determine the format for these cases was to ask residents from around the country to weigh in. Overwhelmingly, the residents said that they would prefer a concise, point-by-point presentation of the Essential Facts of each case in an easy-to-read, bulleted format. This approach is easy on exhausted eyes and provides a quick review of Pearls and Pitfalls as information is absorbed during repeated study sessions. We worked hard to choose cases that could be presented well in this format, recognizing the limitations inherent in reproducing high-quality images in print. Unlike the authors of other case-based radiology review books, we removed the guesswork by providing clear annotations and descriptions for all images. In our opinion, there is nothing worse than being unable to locate a subtle finding on a poorly reproduced image even after one knows the final diagnosis.

The electronic cases expand on the printed book and provide a comprehensive review of the entire subspecialty. Thousands of cases are strategically designed to increase the resident's knowledge by providing exposure to additional case examples—from basic to advanced—and by exploring "Aunt Minnie's," unusual diagnoses, and variability within a single diagnosis. The search engine gives the resident a fighting chance to find the Holy Grail by creating individualized, daily study lists that are not limited by factors such as a radiology subsection. For example, tailor today's study list to cases involving tuberculosis and include cases in every subspecialty and every system of the body. Or study only thoracic cases, including those with links to cardiology, nuclear medicine, and pediatrics. Or study only musculoskeletal cases. The choice is yours.

As enthusiastic partners in this project, we started small and, with the encouragement, talent, and guidance of Tim Hiscock at Thieme, continued to raise the bar in our effort to assist residents in tackling the daunting task of assimilating massive amounts of information. We are passionate about continuing this journey, hoping to expand the cases in our electronic series, adapt cases based on direct feedback from residents, and increase the features intended for board review and self-assessment. As the American Board of Radiology converts its certifying examinations to an electronic format, our series will be the one best suited to meet the needs of the next generation of overworked and exhausted residents in radiology.

*Jonathan Lorenz, MD*
*Hector Ferral, MD*
*Chicago, IL*

# Preface

The gastrointestinal (GI) component of the RadCases series covers the spectrum of GI diagnosis using all related modalities, including computed tomography, magnetic resonance imaging, fluoroscopic studies, and ultrasound. In the home stretch of your exam preparation, you should concentrate on cases most likely to appear on the boards and then repeatedly prime the core concepts pertinent to those cases. This book provides those concepts in a single, concise, accurate, and comprehensive collection of essential cases presented with high-quality images and clear annotations of normal anatomy and pathology. In many cases, more than one diagnosis is present within a single case to test your eye and avoid the tendency for critical details to be missed as a result of satisfaction-of-search phenomenon. In addition, throughout the 100 print cases and 150 additional web-based cases, various versions of critical diagnoses are repeated to better prepare you for the unknown cases on the actual board exam. The electronic component of this book consists of sortable, high-resolution cases to help you tailor study sessions to your needs.

This compilation of cases is the result of an intense search for the best examples of diagnoses in gastrointestinal radiology, and I am confident that complete mastery of gastrointestinal radiology will prepare you well for case conferences, clinical work, and radiology board exams.

# Acknowledgments

I would like to thank Timothy Hiscock at Thieme Publishers for his expertise, patience, and encouragement. In addition, I owe a debt of gratitude to the chairman of the Radiology Department at the University of Chicago, Richard Baron, for his continued encouragement and support, and to the rest of the radiologists of the body imaging section of the University of Chicago, including Brian Funaki, Aytekin Oto, Arunas Gaspairitis, David Paushter, Michael Vannier, Paul Chang, and Abraham Dachman. Finally, I thank Katy Whipple for her expert technical assistance.

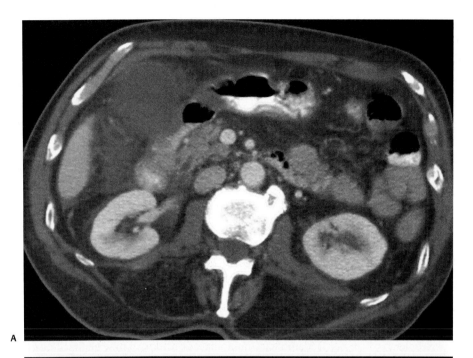

A

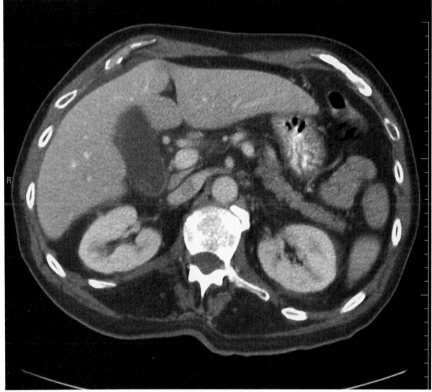

B

## ▪ Clinical Presentation

A 55-year-old diabetic man in the intensive care unit is referred to radiology for fever of unknown origin, leukocytosis, and no significant abdominal pain.

## Imaging Findings

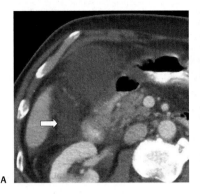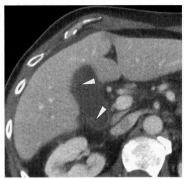

(A) Axial contrast-enhanced computed tomography (CT) image shows a thickened and indistinct gallbladder wall, pericholecystic fluid and edematous fat (*arrow*), gallbladder distension, and no gallstones. (B) Additional axial cut shows linear densities within the gallbladder lumen, consistent with sloughed intraluminal mucosal membranes (*arrowheads*).

## Differential Diagnosis

- *Acute cholecystitis:* This is indicated by pericholecystic fat stranding and the clinical presentation. As no gallstones are visible, the findings suggest acalculous cholecystitis (AC). Sloughed mucosal membranes within the gallbladder indicate gangrenous cholecystitis.
- *Adjacent inflammation or infection from diverticulitis, hepatitis, pancreatitis, or peptic ulcer disease:* This can secondarily involve the gallbladder or mimic acute cholecystitis.

## Essential Facts

- AC is inflammation of the gallbladder without gallstones and represents only 5% of cases of cholecystitis. Untreated AC progresses rapidly and has a high risk of mortality.
- Predisposing conditions include diabetes, malignancy, burn injury, recent surgery or trauma, cardiac disease, positive-pressure ventilation, and total parenteral nutrition.
- The clinical presentation may differ from that of calculous cholecystitis in that the severity of disease may be out of proportion to the severity of right upper quadrant pain. Some patients are pain-free despite leukocytosis and fever.
- Severe presentations of AC:
  - Gangrenous cholecystitis may occur with calculous or acalculous cholecystitis and is an ominous, advanced stage caused by secondary ischemic necrosis; look for sloughed membranes, intramural/intraluminal gas, an irregular/absent gallbladder wall, and abscess.
  - Emphysematous cholecystitis may occur with calculous or acalculous cholecystitis and is an ominous condition usually caused by *Escherichia coli* and *Klebsiella*. Fifty percent of cases occur in the setting of diabetes, and the characteristic finding is intramural gas.
- Treatment options include percutaneous cholecystostomy (usually the first-line and definitive treatment for AC), surgical cholecystectomy, and endoscopic nasobiliary drain for suboptimal surgical or radiologic candidates.

## Other Imaging Findings

- Hepatobiliary iminodiacetic acid scan may be first-line or in cases equivocal for AC on CT or ultrasound; a positive study shows nonvisualization of technetium technetium-99m iminodiacetic acid within the gallbladder after 4 hours or after intravenous morphine.
- Ultrasound is the best modality for the evaluation of cholecystitis, although AC is often diagnosed by CT during the work-up of chronically ill patients for fever of unknown origin. Look for absent stones, sludge, luminal distension, pericholecystic fluid, and wall thickening that is hyperemic by power Doppler.

## ✓ Pearls & ✗ Pitfalls

- ✓ Systemic diseases such as hypoproteinemia or organ failure (liver, renal, heart) can mimic imaging findings of acute AC.
- ✓ Calculous cholecystitis may present on ultrasound with the wall-echo-shadow sign, indicating large stones against the gallbladder wall.
- ✓ Xanthogranulomatous cholecystitis typically occurs in the setting of chronic calculous cholecystitis and can be confused with gallbladder carcinoma; this is a destructive, inflammatory process often associated with mural thickening with hypodense intramural nodules (infiltrated lipid-laden macrophages).
- ✗ A low threshold for imaging in high-risk patients and for cholecystostomy in equivocal cases is required because AC is life-threatening and rapidly progressing despite the mild outward clinical signs.

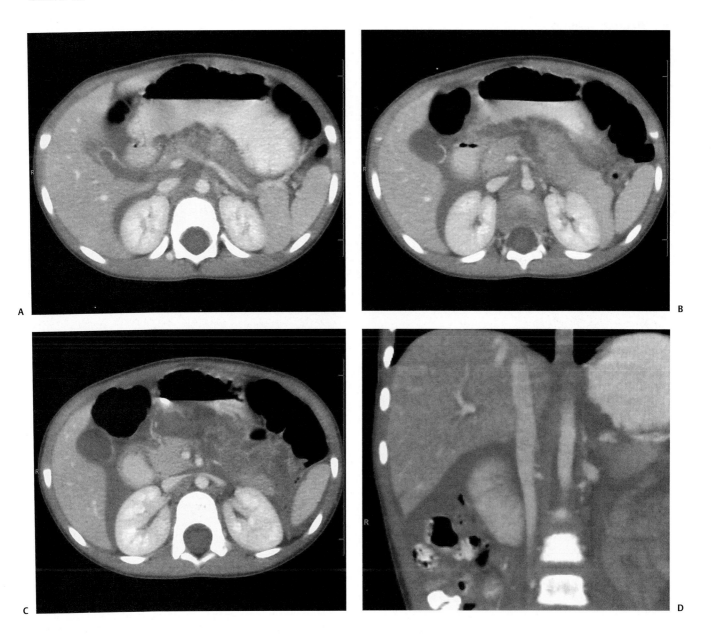

## ■ Clinical Presentation

A 3-year-old boy presents to the emergency department after a motor vehicle accident.

## ■ Imaging Findings

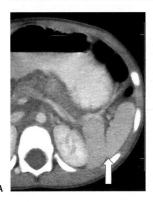 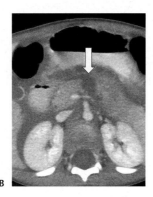 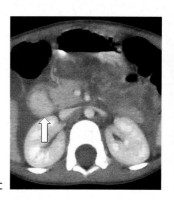 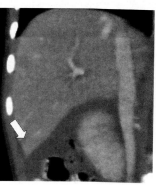

**(A)** Infused computed tomography (CT) shows a linear hypodensity (*arrow*) involving the spleen that is smoothly encapsulated at its margins and associated with no perisplenic fluid, consistent with a splenic cleft. **(B)** More caudal image shows an irregularly marginated hypodense lesion (*arrow*) in the pancreatic neck and head, enlargement of the more distal pancreas, and retroperitoneal fluid, indicating pancreatic transection. **(C)** More caudal image shows contrast within the second portion of the duodenum (*arrow*), which appears mildly dilated. Duodenal injury should be considered but is not clearly identified. **(D)** Coronal reformatted image shows a 1-cm linear hypodensity (*arrow*) involving the right lobe of the liver with perihepatic fluid, consistent with a small laceration.

## ■ Differential Diagnosis

• ***Pancreatic laceration, hepatic laceration, and splenic cleft:*** This is the only diagnosis, given the irregularly marginated, low-density linear defect in the pancreas; the short, linear, hypodense lesion in the right lobe of the liver; and the encapsulated, smooth margins of the splenic defect.

## ■ Essential Facts

• Pancreatic injury is common in blunt trauma cases because of the fixed nature of the pancreas in the retroperitoneum and the tendency for crush injury of the body against the vertebral column to occur.
• Pancreatic laceration is the most prominent finding because the pancreas is nearly transected. Abridged descriptions of grades A to C:
  • Grade A: < 50% thickness laceration or focal pancreatitis
  • Grade B: > 50% laceration of the body or tail (B1) or transection of the body or tail (B2)
  • Grade C: > 50% laceration of the head (C1) or transection of the head (C2)
• CT findings in pancreatic injury include linear, hypodense lacerations; pancreatic enlargement; inhomogeneous enhancement; peripancreatic fluid; blood and fat stranding; and thickened pararenal fascia.
• Associated injuries to the biliary tree, gallbladder, kidney, spleen, liver, and duodenum are common.
• Complications of pancreatic injury include pancreatitis, pseudocyst, hemorrhage, and abscess.
• Hepatic laceration in this case is much more subtle because it is only grade I. Abridged descriptions of grades I to VI:
  • Grade I: < 1 cm parenchymal depth

• Grade II: 1 to 3 cm parenchymal depth
• Grade III: > 3 cm parenchymal depth
• Grade IV: 25 to 75% of hepatic lobe or 1 to 3 Couinaud segments within a single lobe
• Grade V: 75% of hepatic lobe or > 3 Couinaud segments within a single lobe and/or juxtavenous hepatic injuries (retrohepatic caval or hepatic venous avulsion)
• Grade VI: hepatic avulsion

## ■ Other Imaging Findings

• Endoscopic retrograde cholangiopancreatography or magnetic resonance cholangiopancreatography may be indicated in cases of pancreatic injury to evaluate for commonly associated pancreatic duct and bile duct injuries.
• Hepatobiliary iminodiacetic acid scans may demonstrate commonly associated gallbladder or bile duct injury (obstruction or peritoneal leakage of radioactive tracer).

## ✓ Pearls & ✗ Pitfalls

✓ Splenic cleft or lobulation can mimic a linear laceration, as in this case. For true splenic laceration, look for irregular margination of the hypodense lesion, active bleeding, and perisplenic hematoma.
✗ Multiple injuries are often present in blunt trauma cases, and the satisfaction-of-search phenomenon can have life-threatening consequences!

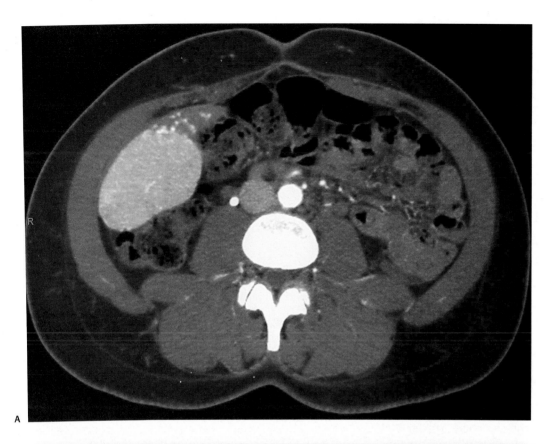

A

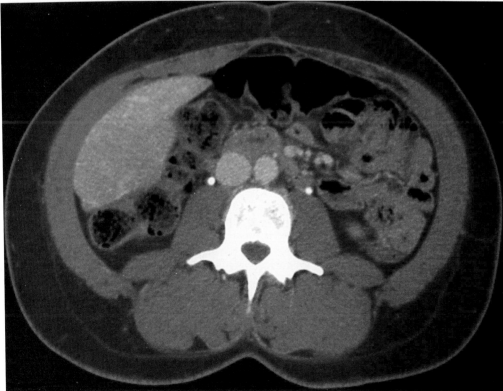

B

## ◼ Clinical Presentation

A 40-year-old woman presents with right upper quadrant pain.

### Imaging Findings

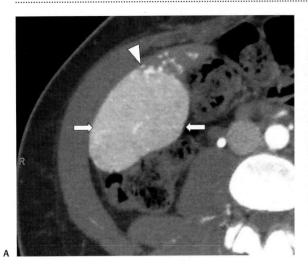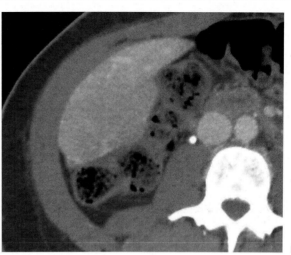

**(A)** Arterial-phase infused computed tomography (CT) shows a solitary, well-circumscribed, enhancing lesion (*arrows*) supplied by adjacent draped arteries (*arrowhead*) originating from the liver. **(B)** Portal venous–phase infused CT: the lesion becomes isoechoic to liver parenchyma on delayed images.

### Differential Diagnosis

- *Hepatic adenoma:* This diagnosis is first on the list for a large, well-circumscribed, solitary lesion with peripherally draped vascular supply in a young woman. Areas of necrosis or hemorrhage would make this diagnosis more convincing and would also produce characteristic heterogeneous enhancement.
- *Focal nodular hyperplasia (FNH):* The lack of a central scar makes FNH less likely, but the central scar is present in only half of FNH cases. The vascular supply is more typically central in FNH.
- *Hepatocellular carcinoma:* Early enhancement makes hepatoma similar to adenoma on imaging; it is less likely in young patients without cirrhosis.

### Essential Facts

- Hepatic adenoma is a benign neoplasm, usually found in young women on oral contraceptives (OCs).
- Associations with hepatic adenoma include glycogen storage disease and steroids.
- Infused CT usually shows a large (mean, 9 cm) and solitary (80%) mass with heterogeneous enhancement due to fat, hemorrhage, and necrosis; a capsule often enhances. Arterial-phase enhancement typically becomes isodense to liver in portal venous phase.
- Hepatic adenomas calcify in 5 to 10% of cases.
- Histopathology shows mostly hepatocytes without portal triads or bile ducts.

- Complications include the common findings of hemorrhage and rupture and the occasional presence of malignant degeneration (to hepatoma).

### Other Imaging Findings

- Technetium-99m sulfur colloid study: adenomas may contain Kupffer cells, resulting in variable uptake.
- Magnetic resonance imaging: adenomas are often hyperintense to liver on T1 and T2 and may drop signal intensity on out-of-phase gradient-echo images because of fatty hepatocytes, glycogen, or hemorrhage.

### ✓ Pearls & ✗ Pitfalls

✓ Adenomas more commonly rupture or hemorrhage compared with FNH.

✓ Adenomas are usually larger than FNH at presentation.

✓ Adenomas are associated with OCs, whereas FNH is not. Stop OCs and reimage later!

✗ Enhancement of adenomas, FNH, and hepatomas may be similar.

✗ Adenomas are typically resected (unlike FNH) because of the risk for degeneration to hepatoma.

✗ Biopsy may be necessary to distinguish adenoma from FNH or hepatoma.

✗ As adenomas are often isodense on delayed infused CT, they may be missed without the performance of quality, multiphase CT.

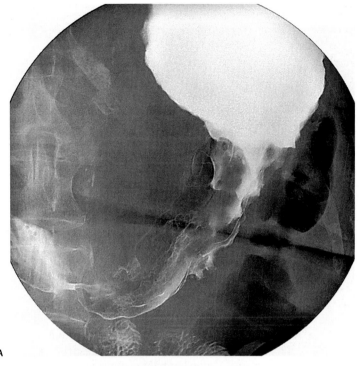

A

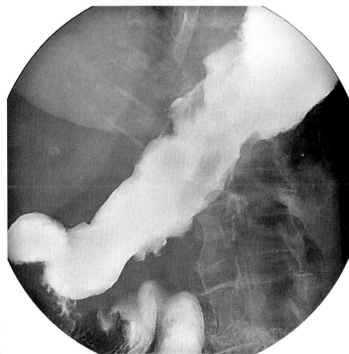

B

## ■ Clinical Presentation

An 82-year-old man presents with midepigastric pain, nausea, and weight loss.

### ■ Imaging Findings

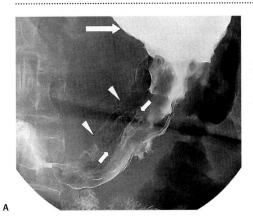
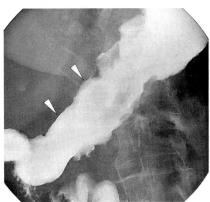

**(A)** Double-contrast study of the body and antrum of the stomach show abnormal lack of distensibility compared with the prominently distended, contrast-filled fundus (*large arrow*). The mucosa is featureless, with distortion of the mucosal pattern in the midbody (*small arrows*) and loss of the areae gastricae along the lesser curve (*arrowheads*). **(B)** Single-contrast study shows no difference in the abnormal tubular constriction of the body and antrum (*arrowheads*).

### ■ Differential Diagnosis

- *Scirrhous carcinoma causing linitis plastica:* This diagnosis is the most common cause of this nonspecific gastric appearance.
- *Lymphoma:* Lymphoma is the second most common cause of linitis plastica. Among the many manifestations of lymphoma, diffuse, circumferential, mural infiltration of the stomach can result in a tubular configuration.
- *Metastatic disease:* Metastatic disease, usually from breast carcinoma, can also cause linitis plastica.
- *Gastritis and peptic ulcer disease:* This option may be severe enough to cause diffuse scarring and lack of distensibility. Consider eosinophilic gastritis, tuberculosis, or corrosive ingestion.

### ■ Essential Facts

- Lack of distensibility of the stomach reproducible on multiple images of an upper gastrointestinal (GI) barium study is highly suggestive of an infiltrative or cicatricial process. Scirrhous carcinoma and gastric lymphoma should be the first considerations.
- Scirrhous carcinoma is an infiltrating gastric carcinoma that classically results in mural rigidity caused by a diffuse desmoplastic reaction. The location is most commonly antral, but the body can be affected, as in this case.
- Gastric lymphoma is the most common presentation of GI lymphoma, and diffuse mural infiltration is the most common manifestation.

### ■ Other Imaging Findings

- Computed tomography may help distinguish gastric carcinoma from lymphoma, although an imaging distinction is often not possible and endoscopic biopsy is required.

- With lymphoma, the lymph nodes are often much bulkier and in remote locations (perirenal, pelvic, chest) because non-Hodgkin lymphoma often presents as a diffuse disease.
- Lymphoma typically causes more marked mural thickening (> 4 cm) and is double the typical thickness of gastric carcinoma.
- Gastric carcinoma is more commonly an ulcerated mass or a polypoid lesion.

### ✓ Pearls & ✗ Pitfalls

- ✓ Radiation enteritis can cause chronic scarring and deformity of any segment of bowel in the radiation portal due to sclerosis of distal arterial branches (endarteritis obliterans). The clinical history is key!
- ✓ Pancreatic carcinoma can infiltrate the stomach and cause rigidity. Look for mass effect and localized invasion (not always present).
- ✓ Crohn disease of the stomach occurs in one-third of patients with Crohn disease and more typically results in a tubular antrum and a narrowed pylorus and duodenum ("ram's horn" sign). Crohn disease causes ulceration, nodularity, a cobblestone configuration, and fistula/fissure formation, and it almost always occurs with ileal and/or colonic involvement.
- ✗ Chronic scarring from peptic ulcer disease can have an appearance similar to that of a desmoplastic reaction from scirrhous carcinoma: a featureless, attenuated lumen. Endoscopy and/or cross-sectional imaging may be performed to make this distinction.

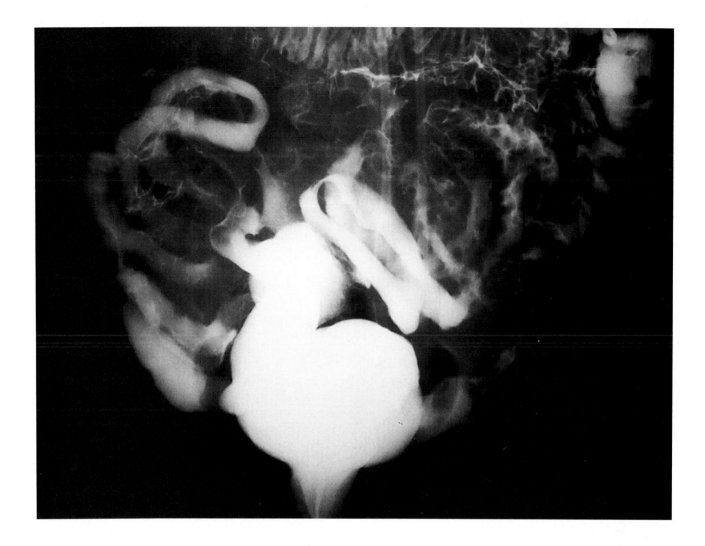

## ■ Clinical Presentation

A 39-year-old presents with severe cramping and watery diarrhea after treatment for acute lymphocytic leukemia.

## ■ Imaging Findings

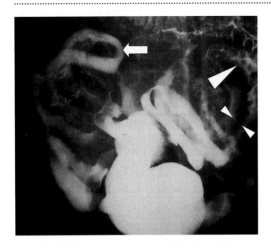

Single-contrast barium study shows diffuse separation of the jejunal loops (*small arrow-heads*) as well as the ileal loops; featureless, ribbonlike ileum (*arrow*) with luminal narrow-ing; and markedly thickened, nodular jejunal folds (*large arrowhead*). The sigmoid colon is also featureless.

## ■ Differential Diagnosis

- ***Graft-versus-host disease (GVHD):*** This diagnosis is indicated by the classic history and imaging findings of diffuse, ribbon-like bowel.
- *Radiation enteritis:* Radiation enteritis is usually more localized as it involves structures within the radiation port, but it may also cause ribbonlike or nodular bowel loops.
- *Infection by cytomegalovirus (CMV) or* Cryptosporidium: This may have a similar appearance and clinical presentation. CMV infection may occur in an immunocompromised host or be secondary to GVHD.

## ■ Essential Facts

- GVHD is marked, multisystemic inflammation usually occurring within 100 days after bone marrow transplant (including autologous!) performed after induction radiation and/or chemotherapy. Acute and chronic forms are observed.
- Locations include the gastrointestinal (GI) tract, lungs, liver, and skin. GVHD of the GI tract is most pronounced in the small bowel and colon, as in this case.
- Pathogenesis is believed to be severe, acute enteritis caused by an immune response mounted by transplanted lymphocytes against the host tissue. This response is made possible by destruction of the host defenses by a combination of induction chemotherapy and immuno-suppressive drugs.
- Barium imaging shows the classic findings demonstrated in this case, including marked fold and mural thickening progressing to featureless, narrowed ileum ("ribbon like" or "toothpastelike") and marked separation of bowel loops. The jejunum is often normal but may show involvement, as in this case, occasionally progressing to featureless bowel.
- Colonic involvement may show a markedly edematous wall, luminal narrowing, occasional ulcerations, and progression to featureless bowel.

- Alternative considerations:
  - Radiation enteritis is the main alternative diagnostic consideration and may cause thickened, fixed, feature-less, separated loops of bowel on barium studies. This entity may have an acute stage of enteritis with severe diarrhea, similar to GVHD, but often presents as sub-acute or chronic enteritis with bowel obstruction and ulceration causing GI bleeding.
  - CMV can superinfect patients with GVHD or primarily infect immunosuppressed patients. Clinical and imaging features of severe CMV enteritis are similar to those of GVHD.

## ■ Other Imaging Findings

- Computed tomography of GVHD may show marked, diffuse small-bowel and colon wall thickening, pneumatosis, and surrounding edema, similar to radiation enteritis.

## ✓ Pearls & ✗ Pitfalls

- ✓ GVHD can be exacerbated by a host of opportunistic infections due to the causative underlying condition of immunocompromise.
- ✓ Moulage pattern of celiac disease is mentioned here only for the characteristic imaging finding of ribbon-like jejunum occurring after long-standing disease. The clinical history should distinguish this entity from GVHD or radiation enteritis.
- ✓ Ulcerative colitis can result in featureless, ahaustral colon, but the small bowel is not affected, and the clinical picture of known, long-standing disease distinguishes this entity.
- ✗ History and disease distribution are critical in the evaluation of patients with barium findings of feature-less, ribbonlike bowel.

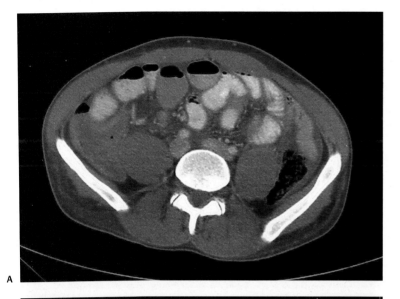

A

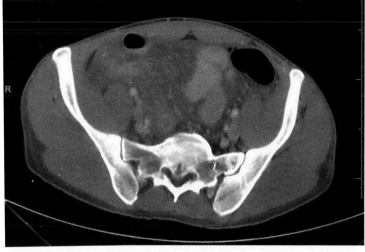

B

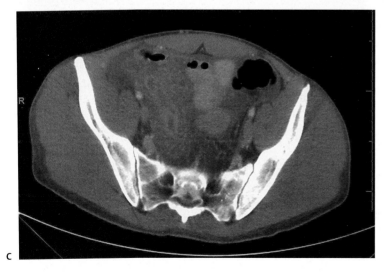

C

## ◼ Clinical Presentation

A 45-year-old man presents with severe pelvic pain.

## ◼ Imaging Findings

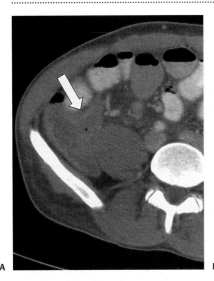
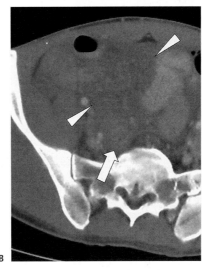
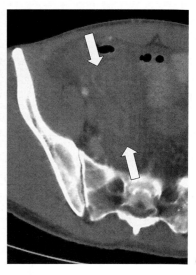

A   B   C

**(A)** Infused abdominal computed tomography (CT) shows thickening of the cecal wall (*arrow*). **(B)** Lower image shows diffuse infiltration of the mesenteric fat (*arrowheads*) within the right lower quadrant (RLQ) and pelvis. A round, enhancing structure (*arrow*) is seen in the pelvis. **(C)** Lower image shows this structure to be tubular (*arrows*), with an enhancing wall and central fluid density.

## ◼ Differential Diagnosis

- **Acute appendicitis:** Acute appendicitis should be the first consideration for a tubular pelvic structure with a thick enhancing wall, mesenteric fat infiltration, and cecal wall thickening.
- *Crohn disease:* Crohn disease may have an identical description to that of acute appendicitis. Both the cecum and the terminal ileum (TI) are commonly involved. The TI may be rigid, thickened, and tubular, like an inflamed appendix. Crohn disease may cause appendicitis in up to 25% of cases. Oral contrast helps distinguish the appendix from the TI.
- *Infectious enteritis:* This may have the same appearance as the previous diagnoses; consider bugs affecting the TI, as in *Yersinia* infection, tuberculosis, and actinomycosis.

## ◼ Essential Facts

- Appendicitis results from obstruction of the lumen of the appendix. The peak age is 10 to 30 years.
- Location may be atypical, including pelvic in a third of cases. Other locations include retroperitoneal in 5% and, less commonly, left-sided appendicitis due to either excessive appendiceal length (mean, 10 cm) or malrotation.
- Appendiceal obstruction may result from lymphoid hyperplasia, appendicolith, tumor, or Crohn disease.
- Clinical presentation varies and may overlap with those of other common infectious processes, including diverticulitis, infectious enteritis, and pelvic inflammatory disease in women. Typical symptoms are RLQ pain, fever, nausea, and vomiting.

- CT appearance varies:
  - Obliteration of the appendix with resultant nonvisualization is the most common appearance by the time patients present to the hospital.
  - Appendiceal diameter ≥ 6 mm and circumferential wall thickening ≥ 2 mm suggest appendicitis.
  - Other possible signs include appendicolith in 25%, mesenteric fat stranding, pericecal abscess, and phlegmon consisting of a mass of soft-tissue and fluid density.

## ◼ Other Imaging Findings

- Ultrasound may show a distended, fluid-filled, noncompressible appendix that appears tubular or target-like, with the dimensions previously described. Periappendiceal fluid or phlegmon may be present.
- Barium filling the appendix to its bulbous tip rules out appendicitis but is seen in only a third of cases.

## ✓ Pearls & ✗ Pitfalls

- ✓ Appendicolith makes the diagnosis. If the remainder of the findings are subtle or indeterminate, an appendicolith and a high level of clinical suspicion are enough to send patients to the operating room.
- ✓ In women, pelvic appendicitis and tubo-ovarian abscess may be indistinguishable both clinically and on imaging studies, particularly when a normal appendix is not visualized.
- ✗ Mesenteric adenitis may mimic appendicitis and typically presents with isolated RLQ adenopathy, occasionally with cecal wall thickening. Features that distinguish this entity include a normal appendix and adenopathy greater than the mild adenopathy typical with appendicitis.

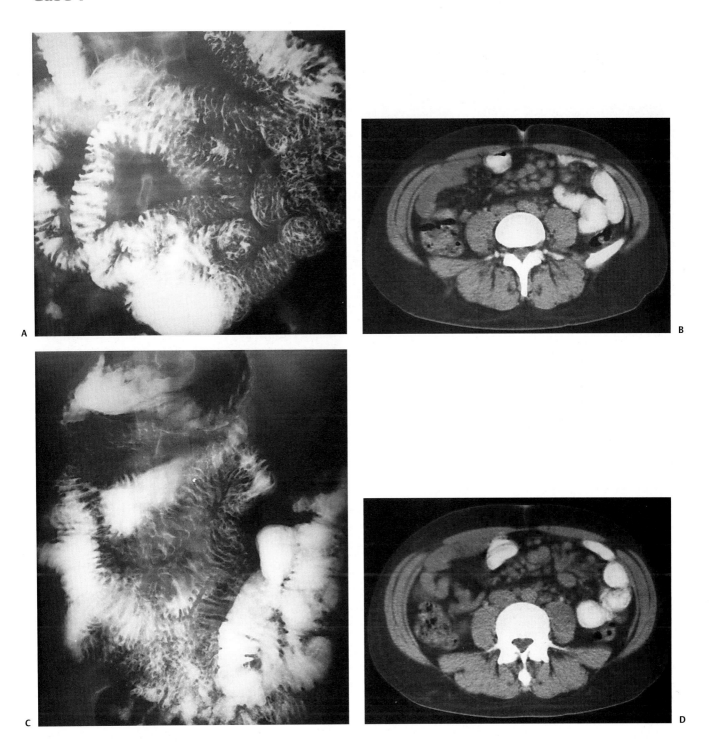

## Clinical Presentation

A 52-year-old man presents with severe diarrhea.

## ■ Imaging Findings

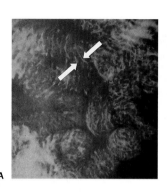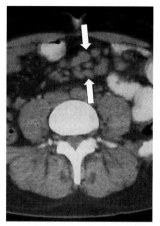

**(A)** Small-bowel (SB) follow-through study shows diffusely thickened, irregular, nodular jejunal folds (*between arrows*). **(B)** Axial computed tomography (CT) after oral contrast shows a cluster of enlarged mesenteric lymph nodes in the midabdomen (*arrows*).

## ■ Differential Diagnosis

- **Mycobacterium avium-intracellulare *(MAI) infection:*** Irregular, nodular fold thickening, adenopathy, and diarrhea all point to MAI infection as the correct diagnosis.
- *Whipple disease:* Whipple disease can present with similar imaging and clinical findings, but with fatty, bulkier adenopathy.
- *Lymphoma:* Lymphoma can cause diffuse fold thickening, but typically the adenopathy will be more prominent.

## ■ Essential Facts

- This case reviews the differential diagnosis for nodular, thickened folds of SB with lymphadenopathy.
- MAI infection, also known as pseudo-Whipple disease, is caused by an acid-fast bacillus and is often seen as a late complication of acquired immunodeficiency syndrome (CD4 count < 100/mm$^3$), which differentiates this entity from Whipple disease.
  - Clinical presentation is diarrhea due to malabsorption.
  - Imaging findings may include a granular surface with thickened walls on enteroclysis (classic finding, most pronounced in the jejunum), in addition to mesenteric and retroperitoneal lymphadenopathy on CT (classic finding, often with low attenuation). Hepatosplenomegaly may be present.
- Whipple disease is caused by *Tropheryma whippelii.*
  - Clinical presentation is diarrhea due to malabsorption.
  - Imaging findings include mucosal micronodularity on enteroclysis (usually jejunal) and bulky lymph nodes with low attenuation (fatty) on CT. Hepatosplenomegaly may be present.
  - Imaging-guided biopsy of the enlarged lymph nodes can establish the diagnosis by demonstrating periodic acid–Schiff-positive glycoprotein granules.

## ■ Other Imaging Findings

- Gallium scan of MAI pneumonia may show increased uptake in lungs
- CT may show microabscesses in the liver and spleen appearing as small, low-density lesions.

## ✓ Pearls & ✗ Pitfalls

- ✓ Normal SB fold density is > 5 folds per inch in the jejunum and 2 to 4 folds per inch in the ileum.
- ✓ SB fold thickening should be distinguished as localized (segmental) versus diffuse and as straight versus irregular/nodular.
- ✓ Diffuse thickening may be due to MAI infection, Whipple disease, lymphoma, lymphangiectasia, hypoproteinemia, amyloidosis, or mastocytosis. Crohn disease uncommonly causes diffuse fold thickening.
- ✓ Nodular folds may be due to eosinophilic gastroenteritis, amyloidosis, MAI infection, Whipple disease, lymphangiectasia, or lymphoma.
- ✓ Localized thickening may be due to neoplasm, ischemia, hemorrhage, Crohn disease, or infection and is often differentiable by location: *Cryptosporidium* and *Giardia* in the proximal small bowel and jejunum, and *Mycobacterium tuberculosis* in the terminal ileum.
- ✓ Adenopathy may be associated with SB MAI infection, Whipple disease, lymphoma, Crohn disease, or amyloidosis.

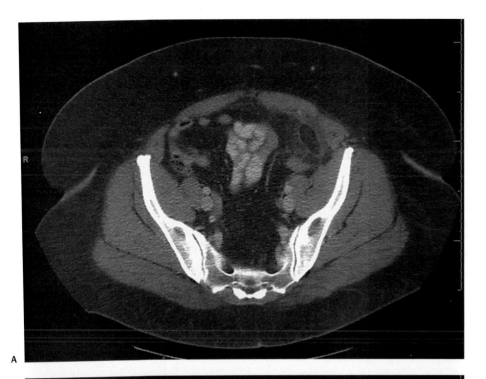

A

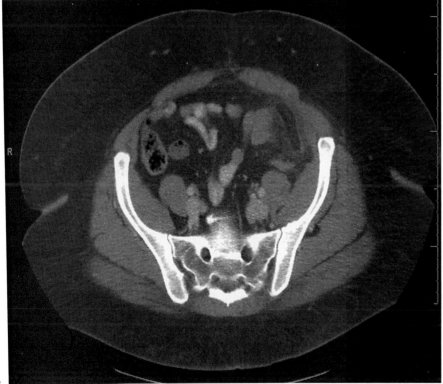

B

## ■ Clinical Presentation

A 50-year-old woman presents to the emergency department with the recent onset of left lower quadrant pain.

## ■ Imaging Findings

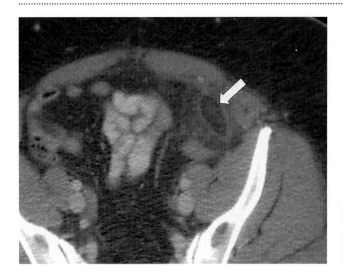

Enhanced axial computed tomography (CT) shows a fatty structure anterior to the sigmoid colon surrounded by a hyperdense rim (*arrow*) and edematous fat stranding. A central focus of increased density within this structure represents infarcted vein due to torsion of the vascular pedicle of the epiploic appendage, which is the root cause of this condition.

## ■ Differential Diagnosis

- *Acute epiploic appendagitis:* This usually presents as an oval fatty structure adjacent to the anterior sigmoid colon surrounded by a hyperdense ring.
- *Omental infarction:* This can also present as a larger structure in the right lower quadrant with a heterogeneous whirl of stranded fat between the abdominal wall and ascending/transverse colon. However, it displays no hyperdense ring in most cases.
- *Acute inflammatory conditions:* Focal inflammatory conditions are unlikely in this case, but in some cases of apparent epiploic appendagitis, diverticulitis or appendicitis should be considered.

## ■ Essential Facts

- Acute epiploic appendagitis is torsion and resulting inflammation of an epiploic appendage (peritoneal fatty pouches arising from the serosal surface of the colon). The vascular pedicle from the colon to the appendage is occluded by torsion, causing acute ischemia.
- Locations: adjacent to sigmoid colon > descending colon > ascending colon
- Risk factors include obesity and hernia.
- Presentation is typically acute lower quadrant pain mimicking diverticulitis or appendicitis and is usually in men 30 to 50 years of age.
- Prognosis: usually self-limited; epiploic appendagitis is rarely associated with peritonitis, abscess, or bowel obstruction.
- Treatment is antiinflammatory medications, except in rare, complicated cases requiring surgery for peritonitis or percutaneous drainage of an abscess.
- Fat-containing tumors can rarely mimic epiploic appendagitis: consider liposarcoma, dermoid, angiomyolipoma, and metastasis in some cases.

## ■ Other Imaging Findings

- CT shows an oval structure abutting the colon (usually sigmoid), near fat density, < 5 cm with surrounding fat stranding. Colon wall is usually normal. A central focus of high density may be present, indicating venous thrombosis from torsion, as in this case.
- Barium enema is usually normal.

## ✓ Pearls & ✗ Pitfalls

- ✓ Normally, epiploic appendages are not visible by CT unless inflamed and surrounded by edematous fat.
- ✓ Imaging findings of epiploic appendagitis are distinguished from those of similar entities by size (< 5 cm), location (usually perisigmoidal), the absence of colon wall thickening, and the presence of a hyperdense ring.
- ✓ The mesenteric lipodystrophy form of retractile mesenteritis is mostly fat necrosis but is distinguished from epiploic appendagitis by association with the bowel mesentery. The fat plane around the involved mesenteric vessels is called the "fat ring" sign but typically has no hyperdense ring.
- ✗ Acute epiploic appendagitis may lead to unnecessary surgery by mimicking the clinical presentation and imaging appearance of acute abdomen, tumors, and inflammatory conditions.

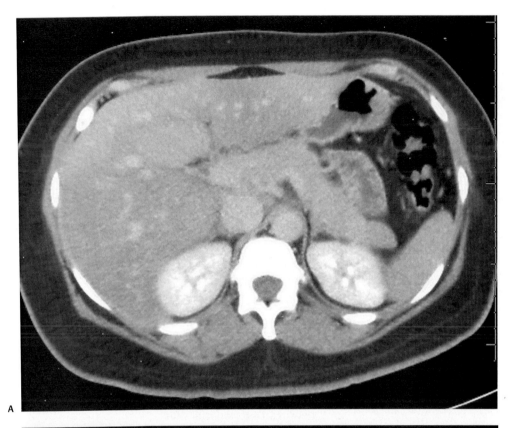

A

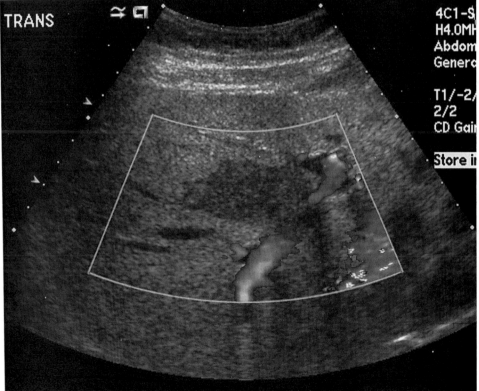

B

## ■ Clinical Presentation

A 54-year-old man presents with vague abdominal symptoms and weight loss.

### ▧ Imaging Findings

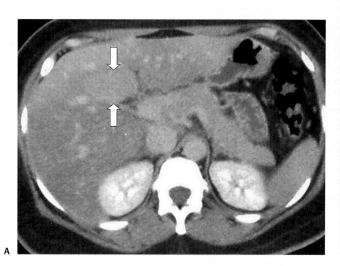

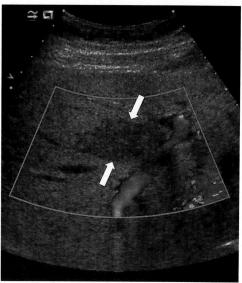

**(A)** Infused abdominal computed tomography (CT) shows hypoattenuation of the liver sparing an ovoid portion (*arrows*) of the medial segment of the left lobe. **(B)** Ultrasound shows this ovoid region (*arrows*) to be adjacent to the portal vein, well defined, and hypoechoic compared with the remainder of the liver.

### ▧ Differential Diagnosis

- **Focal fatty sparing:** This is the most likely diagnosis for a well-defined, relatively hyperdense region of the medial segment of the left lobe in an otherwise hypodense liver suspicious for hepatic steatosis. The periportal location and absence of mass effect further support this diagnosis.
- *Hepatic tumor:* This is the principal alternative diagnosis for a focal, masslike lesion in the liver; however, the characteristics described above make a tumor extremely unlikely.

### ▧ Essential Facts

- Hepatic steatosis is abnormally increased storage of triglycerides within the hepatocytes due to several postulated factors, such as decreased portal perfusion, congenital and acquired abnormalities of fat metabolism, and perfusion by blood with relatively low insulin levels.
  - Clinical presentation is often asymptomatic (incidental finding). Vague right upper quadrant pain or hepatomegaly may be present.
  - Causes include alcoholism, hepatitis, parenteral nutrition, malnutrition, hyperlipidemia, obesity, diabetes, hepatotoxic drugs such as chemotherapeutic agents, and steroids.
  - CT shows the liver parenchyma to be hypodense compared with the spleen on both noninfused and infused studies. The liver is normally denser than the spleen.
  - Ultrasound shows the liver parenchyma to have increased echogenicity.
- Focal fatty sparing is the relative absence of fatty infiltration in a focal region of the liver, as in this case.

- Causes include regional alterations in portal venous flow or an arterioportal shunt.
- Location may be periportal (especially in the medial segment of the left lobe), adjacent to the falciform ligament, subcapsular, or adjacent to the gallbladder fossa.
- CT shows a well-defined region with density equal to or greater than that of the spleen, characteristic of normal hepatic parenchyma.
- Ultrasound shows this region to be hypoechoic with respect to the fat-infiltrated liver.

### ▧ Other Imaging Findings

- Magnetic resonance imaging detection is based on loss of signal on fat-suppressed images or analysis of chemical shift. Fat infiltration shows isointense signal on in-phase and low signal on out-of-phase studies.

### ✓ Pearls & ✗ Pitfalls

- ✓ Focal fatty infiltration may appear tumorlike because of well-defined regions of fat infiltration within normal liver parenchyma, which is the mirror image of focal fatty sparing.
  - Locations are the same as in focal fatty sparing.
  - CT shows focal, hypodense regions on noninfused and infused studies.
  - Ultrasound shows a focal hyperechoic region.
- ✗ Fatty sparing and infiltration can be focal or multifocal and have a variety of geographic shapes and sizes, making distinction from tumors difficult in some cases.

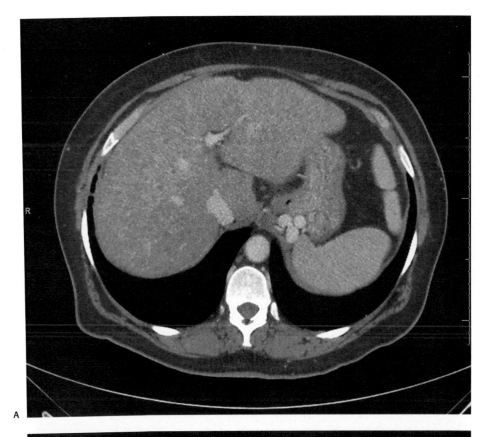

A

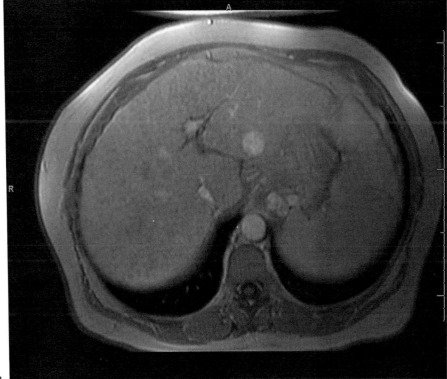

B

## ■ Clinical Presentation

A 63-year-old woman presents with weight loss and nausea.

## ■ Imaging Findings

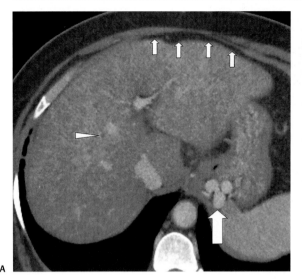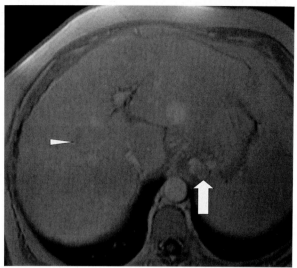

A    B

**(A)** Infused abdominal computed tomography (CT) shows hypertrophy of the left lobe of the liver; reduction of volume of the right lobe; irregular liver contour (*small arrows*); diffusely heterogeneous reduction in liver density (right > left); innumerable small, hypodense parenchymal nodules (*arrowhead*); and a cluster of enhancing structures in the gastric wall, consistent with varices (*large arrow*). **(B)** Infused T1-weighted magnetic resonance imaging (MRI) shows the liver to be abnormally hypointense relative to spleen, resulting from hypointense nodules (*arrowhead*). Mixed signal in gastric varices results from slow, turbulent flow (*arrow*).

## ■ Differential Diagnosis

- **Cirrhosis:** This is the only reasonable item on the differential. It is indicated by classic findings of volume reduction and redistribution to the left lobe, innumerable parenchymal nodules, and gastric varices.
- *Infections:* Infections such as tuberculosis can cause multiple microabscesses in the liver, but the spleen is involved in almost all cases of hepatic microabscesses.

## ■ Essential Facts

- Cirrhosis is the last stage of chronic liver disease, in which the diffuse loss of hepatocytes and extensive fibrosis result in the gross reduction and redistribution of hepatic volume and the formation of regenerative nodules.
- Regenerative nodules contain newly proliferating hepatocytes in an attempt to compensate for loss of liver function.
  - Micronodular or macronodular (depending on whether nodules are > 3 mm or < 3 mm)
  - Benign with premalignant (dysplasia) and malignant (hepatocellular carcinoma) potential
  - CT shows nodules to be hypo- to isodense with and without contrast.
  - MRI shows nodules to be hypointense on T1, T2, and gradient-echo images.
  - Siderotic nodules contain hemosiderin and may be hyperdense on CT and hyperintense on T1 MRI.

## ■ Other Imaging Findings

- Ultrasound of a cirrhotic liver typically shows diffusely echogenic parenchyma with an irregular liver edge, volume loss and redistribution, ascites, varices, loss of the normal hepatic venous triphasic waveform, and increased portal venous pulsatility.

## ✓ Pearls & ✗ Pitfalls

- ✓ Hepatocellular carcinoma is often the principal concern in cirrhotic patients undergoing cross-sectional imaging and is present in 10 to 20% of patients.
  - Suspicious enhancement is maximal during the late arterial phase of contrast infusion on MRI or CT.
  - Suspicious features supporting malignancy include mass effect and vascular invasion.
- ✗ Inhomogeneous enhancement patterns due to focal confluent fibrosis, focal venous obstruction, and arterioportal shunting may lead to overcalling hepatocellular carcinoma in cirrhotic patients.
- ✗ Focal confluent fibrosis is masslike dense fibrosis, often in the medial segment of left lobe or in the anterior right lobe, and is hypo- to isodense on pre- and post-infusion CT.

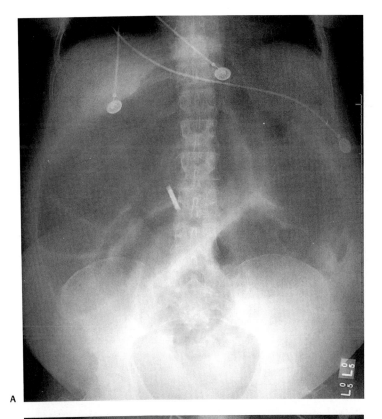

A

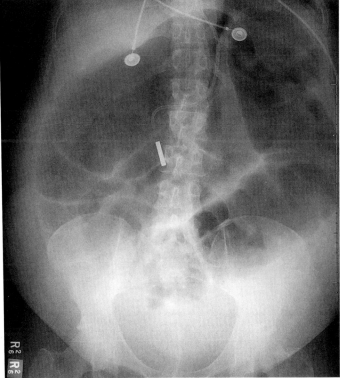

B

## Clinical Presentation

A 56-year-old woman presents with marked abdominal distension. Serial radiographs were obtained during her hospital admission.

### ■ Imaging Findings

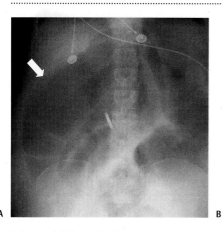 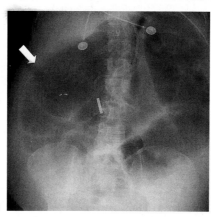 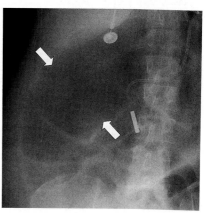

A                                                                      B                                                                      C

**(A)** Frontal abdominal radiograph shows marked dilatation of the ascending, transverse, and descending colon, most pronounced in the proximal colon (*arrow*). There is no air in the rectum, suggesting distal obstruction. **(B)** A later radiograph shows unchanged colonic dilatation (*arrow*) and interval development of a mosaiclike mucosal abnormality with polygonal, raised plaques separated by barium. The patient has no allergies. **(C)** Magnified view of the mucosal abnormality (*arrows*).

### ■ Differential Diagnosis

- **Distal colonic obstruction with colonic urticaria:** Ischemia is the most likely explanation for interval development of this mucosal abnormality.
- *Severe colonic ileus:* This can result in ischemia with colonic urticaria and has a wide array of etiologies.
- *Colitis due to herpes or* Yersinia *infection:* This option can cause colonic urticaria, but here, marked distension precedes any signs of infection, making these entities unlikely.

### ■ Essential Facts

- The key to this case is recognizing the interval development of this radiographically abnormal, reticular mucosal pattern in a markedly dilated colonic segment. Mucosal or, less commonly, submucosal edema is the underlying cause.
- *Colonic urticaria* is a term coined to describe this pattern because it was first discovered in patients having an allergic reaction to medications.
- Colonic obstruction was later associated with the colonic urticaria pattern. This presentation has important clinical implications as it represents mild ischemia of the affected segment, which can progress to frank ulceration and perforation.

- The proximal colon is most commonly affected because of its propensity to dilate the most (cecal diameter of 10 cm heralds rupture). The increased wall tension predisposes the dilated proximal colon to ischemic changes.
- Causes of colonic dilatation that have been associated with colonic urticaria include ileus and distal obstruction resulting from colon carcinoma, diverticulitis, hernia, sigmoid volvulus, or fecal impaction.

### ✓ Pearls & ✗ Pitfalls

- ✓ Crohn disease can cause the colonic urticaria pattern, but this association is uncommon.
- ✓ Absence of air in the rectum suggests distal colonic obstruction rather than colonic ileus, but repeat radiographs in the prone or decubitus positions may rule out distal obstruction by encouraging gas to pass into the rectum.
- ✗ Failure to recognize colonic urticaria can have life-threatening consequences of rapidly advancing bowel ischemia.

# Case 12

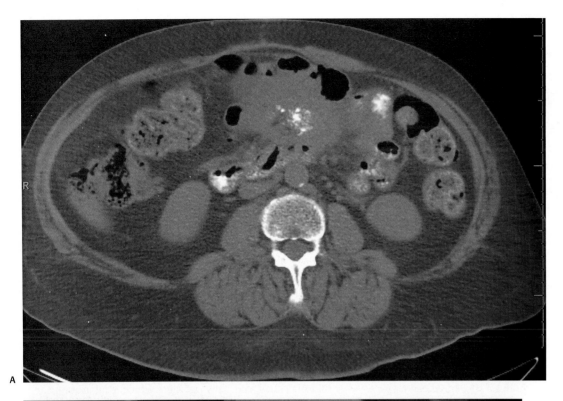

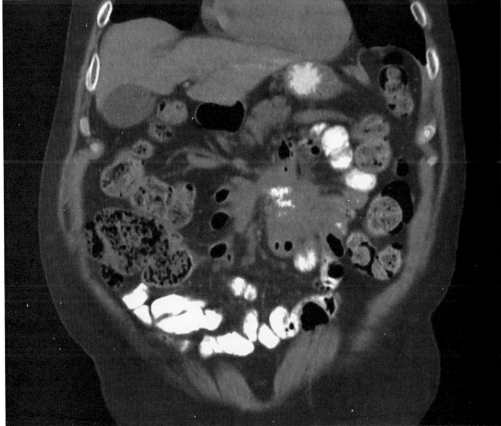

## Clinical Presentation

A 60-year-old man presents with nausea, vomiting, abdominal pain, and fever.

### ■ Imaging Findings

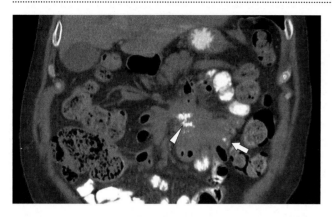

Coronal reformatted computed tomography (CT) shows soft-tissue thickening in the small-bowel mesentery from the superior mesenteric root to the small bowel. Central calcifications (*arrowhead*) and mass effect on small bowel (*arrow*) are noted.

### ■ Differential Diagnosis

- ***Retractile mesenteritis:*** This is strongly suggested by soft-tissue thickening centered at the superior mesenteric root, with central calcifications (typically denser than in carcinoid) extending outward to produce mass effect on the small bowel.
- *Carcinoid:* Desmoplastic reaction of carcinoid metastatic to the mesentery may produce a spoked wheel or star burst pattern of mesenteric thickening and retraction with central calcifications. Hypervascular metastases to liver would suggest this diagnosis over retractile mesenteritis.
- *Metastatic disease:* Other sources of metastatic disease may affect the mesentery.

### ■ Essential Facts

- Retractile mesenteritis is a nonprogressive disease of unknown etiology that may mimic desmoplastic neoplasms.
- A variety of subtypes exist that most likely describe a disease spectrum: mesenteric panniculitis (mostly inflammation), mesenteric lipodystrophy (mostly fat necrosis), and sclerosing mesenteritis (mostly fibrosis).
- In general, retractile mesenteritis:
  - Occurs in decades 5 to 7 with an overall prevalence < 1% but is described in all age groups, including children.
  - Has a small association with lymphoma.
  - Has a nonspecific clinical presentation including nausea, vomiting, fever, abdominal pain, and weight loss.

### ■ Other Imaging Findings

- Small-bowel barium studies may show:
  - Separation of small-bowel loops surrounding the mesenteric root with dense mesenteric calcifications.
  - Small-bowel obstruction, kinking, and tethering.
  - Ischemic bowel (rare) resulting from vascular encasement and mural thickening.
- CT may show the "fat ring" sign, which is fat around mesenteric vessels, as well as variable fat stranding, fat necrosis, and fibrosis.

### ✓ Pearls & ✗ Pitfalls

- ✓ Clinical presentation, histology, and imaging findings of retractile mesenteritis vary as patients pass through a spectrum of inflammation, fat necrosis, and fibrosis.
- ✗ Imaging is nonspecific in the early inflammatory stage (mesenteric fat stranding), and differentiation from carcinoid or other mesenteric metastases may not be possible in some cases.
- ✗ Look for hypervascular metastases to the liver or lymph nodes to favor carcinoid.

# Case 13

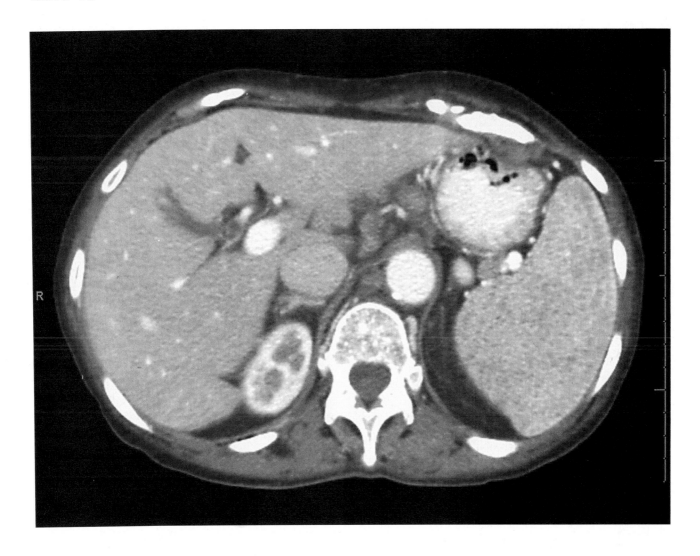

## Clinical Presentation

A 35-year-old woman presents with vague abdominal pain.

## ◼ Imaging Findings

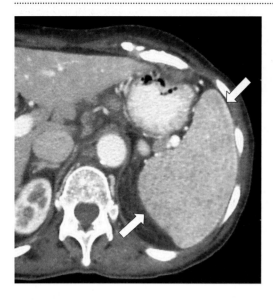

Infused computed tomography shows hypodense micronodules scattered evenly throughout an enlarged spleen (*arrows*).

## ◼ Differential Diagnosis

- *Lymphoma:* This is the most common neoplasm causing the pattern of micronodularity and is the most likely diagnosis for fine, evenly distributed, innumerable nodules, as in this case.
- *Leukemia:* As a second consideration, leukemia can have an identical appearance.
- *Fungal infections:* These can cause hepatosplenic microabscesses, most commonly candidiasis and histoplasmosis.
- *Tuberculosis:* In its disseminated form, tuberculosis can cause hepatosplenic microabscesses.

## ◼ Essential Facts

- The even distribution of fine, tiny, similarly sized micronodules throughout the spleen in this case suggests a neoplastic origin—either lymphoma or leukemia. Infection is still a viable alternative.
- Lymphoma of the spleen and liver can present as focal masses, diffusely scattered nodules, as in this case, or diffuse infiltration and hepatosplenic enlargement without nodularity.
- *Candida albicans* infection can affect the liver and spleen with a micronodular pattern (microabscesses) by disseminating via the hepatic artery and splenic artery. Disseminated *Candida* infection (*Candida* sepsis) typically occurs in immunocompromised hosts.

## ◼ Other Imaging Findings

- Ultrasound of lymphoma of the spleen or liver typically shows lesions that are very hypoechoic and homogeneous, often similar in appearance to cysts.
- Ultrasound of *Candida* microabscesses may show diffuse microabscesses, initially hypoechoic and later presenting as target lesions with an echogenic center (necrosis) surrounded by a hypoechoic rim.
- Magnetic resonance imaging is the most sensitive modality for detecting subtle neoplastic or infectious dissemination in the liver or spleen.

## ✓ Pearls & ✗ Pitfalls

- ✓ Other causes of micronodularity in the spleen typically produce larger and fewer nodules and include metastatic disease, hemangiomas, and lymphangiomas.
- ✓ Sarcoidosis is a rarer granulomatous cause of hepatosplenic micronodularity than fungal or tuberculous infections.
- ✓ Pyogenic infections from bacterial septic embolization are usually cardiac in origin and more typically result in macroabscesses.
- ✗ Patients with lymphoma undergoing chemotherapy and bone marrow transplant are prone to disseminated *Candida* infection due to prolonged neutropenia, making the origin of splenic micronodularity more difficult to determine.
- ✗ The distinction between the micronodularity of lymphoma or leukemia and the microabscesses of *Candida* is often made based on the response to cytotoxic medications versus antifungal medications.

# Case 14

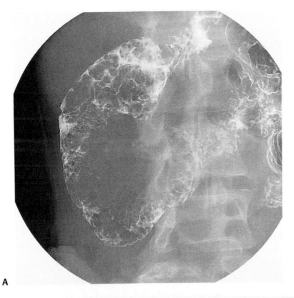

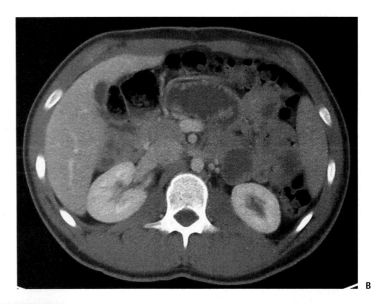

A

B

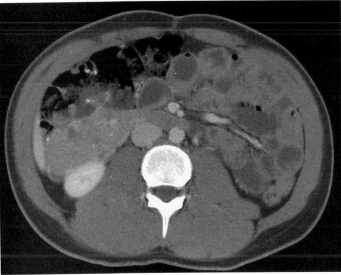

C

## Clinical Presentation

An 18-year-old man presents to the gastroenterology clinic with a history of chronic postprandial nausea, intermittent abdominal pain, and vomiting.

## ■ Imaging Findings

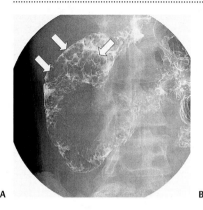
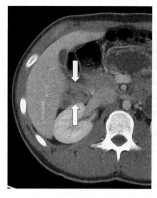
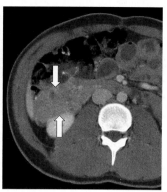

A    B    C

**(A)** Barium study shows multiple, multilobulated, polypoid filling defects (*arrows*) in the first and second portions of the duodenum. **(B)** Contrast-enhanced computed tomography (CT) shows expansion of the duodenum (*arrows*) with soft-tissue masses. **(C)** More caudal image shows marked soft tissue (*arrows*) obliterating the duodenal lumen.

## ■ Differential Diagnosis

- ***Peutz-Jeghers syndrome (PJS; hamartomas):*** This is the most likely diagnosis, given the multiple soft-tissue masses filling the duodenum.
- *Familial adenomatous polyposis (adenomas):* This is a second choice that also may involve the stomach, small bowel, and colon.
- *Juvenile polyposis (hamartomas):* This can occur in the stomach, small bowel, and colon.

## ■ Essential Facts

- PJS is an autosomal-dominant condition with incomplete penetrance in which patients are prone to gastrointestinal (GI) polyps and mucocutaneous pigmentation.
- Multiple hamartomas are usually large and pedunculated, and they present in the stomach, small bowel (most commonly the jejunum and ileum), and colon. The esophagus is spared.
- Occasionally, solitary polyps are the presenting feature.
- Associations include an increased risk for carcinoma of the colon, small bowel, breast, ovaries, testicles, and pancreas.
- Complications include intussusception and GI bleeding that is usually not life-threatening.
- PJS is associated with an increased risk for GI adenomas and adenocarcinomas at a younger age than is typical for these neoplasms.
- Treatment is endoscopic or surgical excision of polyps. If necessary because of marked involvement or complications, symptomatic segments of bowel are resected, sparing as much as possible.
- Additional causes of gastric polyps:
  - Cronkhite-Canada syndrome causes hyperplastic inflammatory polyps and is mostly associated with loss of hair and nails as well as hyperpigmentation.
  - Cowden syndrome causes hamartomas and may occur in the entire GI tract, tongue, and skin.

## ■ Other Imaging Findings

- Small-bowel barium study may show obstruction or a "coiled spring" appearance of intussusception.
- CT may appear as a large, consolidated mass due to multiple, large polyps confined to the duodenal lumen, as in this case.

## ✓ Pearls & ✗ Pitfalls

✓ Non-neoplastic causes of multiple small-bowel polypoid filling defects include nodular lymphoid hyperplasia (smaller than those in this case), Behçet syndrome (ulcerated), amyloidosis (often large), Crohn disease (large or filiform), and hemangiomas.

✓ Neoplastic causes include lymphoma (variable), neurofibromatosis (large, eccentric), lipomas, and metastases (breast, lung, and melanoma).

✓ Polypoid lipomatosis of the small bowel is easily distinguished by the CT finding of fat density within the associated lesions.

✓ GI neoplasms of PJS often occur distant from the site of the hamartomas, suggesting an association with PJS that is not caused by malignant degeneration of PJS hamartomas.

✓ Severe colic with a relatively sudden onset suggests intussusception!

✗ Severe duodenitis or lymphoma with marked mural thickening and obliteration of the lumen can mimic polyposis, and vice versa.

✗ Intraluminal debris/food can mimic polyposis.

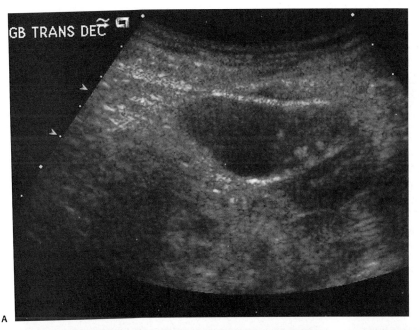

A

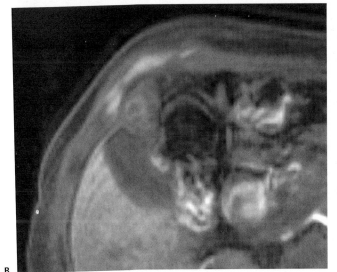

B

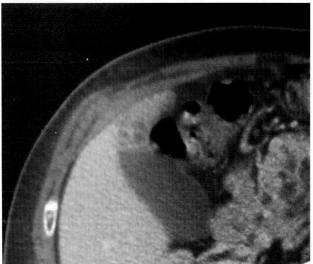

C

## ■ Clinical Presentation

.................................................................................................................................................................

A 53-year-old woman presents with vague abdominal pain.

### ▰ Imaging Findings

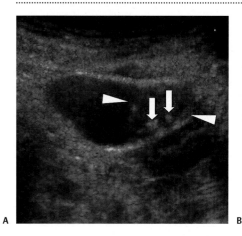
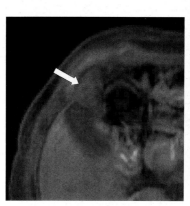
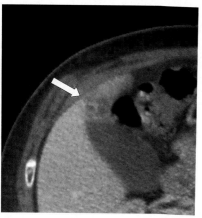

A            B            C

**(A)** Ultrasound shows a focal mass (*arrowheads*) in the fundus of the gallbladder (GB) with internal echogenic foci (*arrows*) without reverberation artifact. There is associated mural thickening. **(B)** Postinfusion T1 magnetic resonance imaging (MRI) shows the mass (*arrow*) to be focal and heterogeneous in signal intensity. The majority of the mass is similar to liver parenchyma except for central regions of low signal intensity. **(C)** Contrast-enhanced computed tomography (CT) shows the mass (*arrow*) to enhance similarly to liver parenchyma and to contain central, nonenhancing, cystic-appearing foci with a density similar to that of the GB lumen.

### ▰ Differential Diagnosis

- **Focal adenomyomatosis:** Given the GB wall thickening and an enhancing, masslike fundal structure with internal, nonenhancing (on CT and MRI), echogenic components, focal adenomyomatosis is the most likely diagnosis.
- *GB adenocarcinoma:* This option should be entertained for any masslike lesion in the GB with enhancing components.
- *Metastasis:* Usually melanoma, it can affect the GB and have central regions of necrosis.
- *Polyp:* Adenomatous polyps are uncommon and more typically appear as smaller (< 2 cm), solitary polyps. Cholesterol polyps are more common and present as intraluminal masses.

### ▰ Essential Facts

- Hyperplastic cholecystosis describes benign tissue proliferation affecting the GB. Subtypes include adenomyomatosis and cholesterolosis, each without malignant potential.
- Adenomyomatosis is mural hyperplasia of the muscular layer and epithelial mucosa with the development of characteristic, mucosa-lined diverticula, called Rokitansky-Aschoff sinuses (RASs), containing sludge, cholesterol crystals, or stones.
- Affects any age; found in 5% of resected GBs
- Types:
  - Focal usually occurs in the fundus, may be crescentic or masslike, and is most common.
  - Segmental usually occurs in the body and may be annular constricting.
  - Diffuse involves most of the GB.

- Clinical presentation: adenomyomatosis is usually asymptomatic and incidental but occasionally presents with pain and may present with gallstones.
- Imaging findings typically include enhancing mural thickening. In addition:
  - Ultrasound shows immobile, echogenic RASs. If cholesterol crystals are present, short comet tail reverberation artifacts may be seen (not present in this case but highly specific).
  - CT shows low-density RASs ("rosary" sign is enhancing RAS mucosa surrounded by nonenhancing muscle).
  - MRI shows intramural RASs that are nonenhancing, with low signal intensity on T1 and high signal intensity on T2 ("pearl necklace" sign of multiple, bright RASs).
- Treatment is not required in most cases. Pain or indeterminate imaging findings may necessitate cholecystectomy.

### ▰ Other Imaging Findings

- Positron emission tomography shows positive fluorodeoxyglucose uptake for GB carcinoma and other benign and malignant neoplasms, but negative uptake for adenomyomatosis and cholesterol polyps.

### ✓ Pearls & ✗ Pitfalls

- ✓ Cholesterolosis is cholesterol and triglyceride deposits in the lamina propria ("strawberry" GB).
- ✗ This case was associated with pain and was quite masslike on imaging studies without the specific sign of comet tail artifact; thus, resection was performed and the pathology was confirmed.

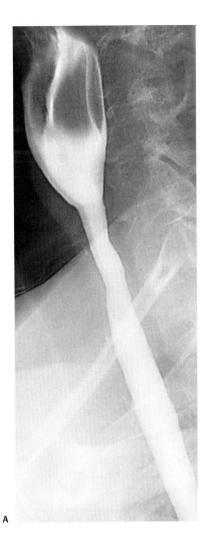 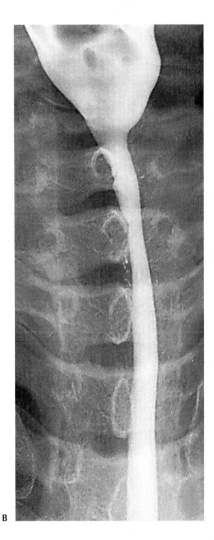 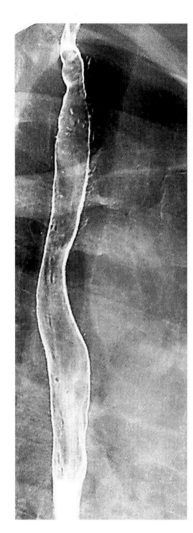

A  B  C

## ▨ Clinical Presentation

A 52-year-old woman presents with heartburn and dysphagia.

## ■ Imaging Findings

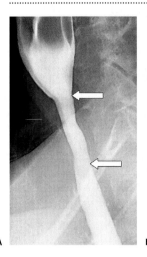
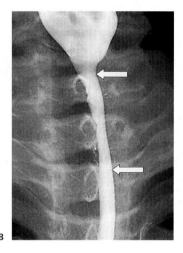
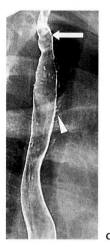

**(A,B)** Single-contrast esophagograms show circumferential narrowing (*arrows*) of the cervical esophagus with a smooth transition to normal-caliber esophagus. This finding persists on both left anterior oblique (A) and frontal (B) projections. **(C)** Double-contrast study again shows narrowing (*arrow*) of the cervical esophagus. Multiple small outpouchings (*arrowhead*) of barium in the proximal esophagus are consistent with intramural pseudodiverticulosis.

## ■ Differential Diagnosis

- **Barrett stricture:** This classically occurs in the middle to upper esophagus and may be associated with intramural pseudodiverticulosis, as seen in this case.
- *Radiation injury from mediastinal irradiation:* This occurs in the distribution of the radiation port. Patients with upper lobe, high mediastinal, or cervical malignancy may be at risk for this complication.
- *Skin diseases:* Epidermolysis bullosa or benign pemphigoid may cause middle to upper strictures.

## ■ Essential Facts

- Esophageal strictures may be diffuse or focal. Focal strictures are best categorized as proximal, middle, or distal for diagnostic purposes.
- Proximal esophageal strictures are the focus of this case and most commonly occur as a result of Barrett esophagus. Depending on the clinical history, other considerations are radiation therapy, caustic ingestion, drug ingestion, and tumors.
- Clinical presentation is usually dysphagia.
- Barrett esophagus is metaplasia of the epithelium from squamous to columnar caused by reflux esophagitis.
  - Malignant degeneration (adenocarcinoma) occurs in 10%.
  - Mucosal ulceration may precede metaplasia.
  - Upper to middle strictures are most commonly Barrett strictures, but Barrett strictures are more common in the distal esophagus near the squamocolumnar junction. Strictures tend to be long, smoothly marginated, circumferential, and tapered.
  - Reticular mucosal pattern on double-contrast barium studies typically extends distal to the proximal esophageal stricture and may indicate a higher risk for malignant degeneration.

## ■ Other Imaging Findings

- Technetium-99m pertechnetate study may show esophageal uptake in Barrett due to epithelial metaplasia.

## ✓ Pearls & ✗ Pitfalls

- ✓ Radiation injury results in acute, ischemic esophagitis and delayed (> 4 months), smoothly marginated, tapered, circumferential strictures.
- ✓ Caustic ingestion leads to mucosal injury and delayed (1–3 months) strictures that may be segmental or run the entire length of the esophagus. These strictures may be mild to severe and often occur in the upper to middle esophagus.
- ✓ A tumor such as metastatic lymphadenopathy can cause circumferential narrowing of the esophageal lumen, but more typically at the level of the aorta rather than the proximal cervical esophagus.
- ✓ Drugs may cause esophageal strictures at locations of esophageal indentation by normal structures such as the aortic arch or left main bronchus. Offending agents include the tetracycline family, potassium chloride, and nonsteroidal antiinflammatory drugs.
- ✓ Intramural pseudodiverticulosis of the esophagus:
  - Represents barium within dilated mucous excretory glands.
  - Rarely occurs in a normal esophagus.
  - Is most commonly associated with benign inflammatory conditions and rarely seen with malignant strictures.
  - Is often present with *Candida*, but the nature of this relationship is unclear.
  - Is associated with alcohol abuse and diabetes.

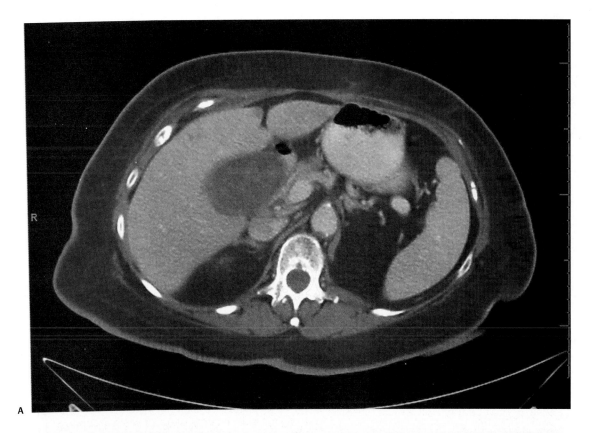

A

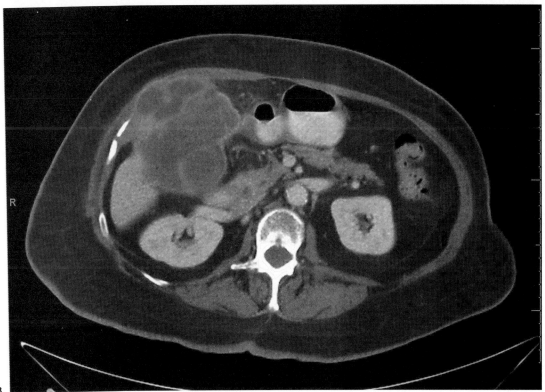

B

## ■ Clinical Presentation

A 69-year-old woman presents with right upper quadrant pain.

### ■ Imaging Findings

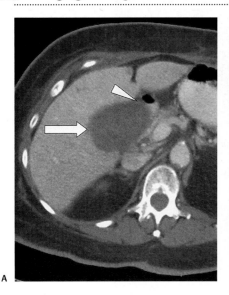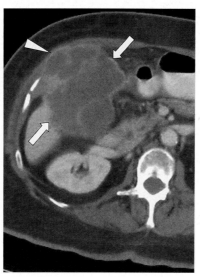

(A) Contrast-enhanced computed tomography shows a multilobular soft-tissue mass occupying most of the lumen of the gallbladder (GB). The GB wall is thickened (*arrow*) and compressing the adjacent duodenum (*arrowhead*). (B) A more caudal image shows a multiloculate cystic mass (*arrows*) surrounding the thickened GB, which is seen posteromedially. This mass may be invading the abdominal wall musculature (*arrowhead*).

### ■ Differential Diagnosis

- *GB adenocarcinoma:* A noncalcified, multilobular mass effacing the GB lumen, GB wall thickening, and an exophytic mass involving the GB and invading the abdominal wall are all features of GB carcinoma.
- *Xanthogranulomatous cholecystitis (XGC):* A multiloculated mass involving the GB and invading the abdominal wall is suspicious for this entity. A more characteristic appearance would include hypodense nodules in the GB wall and stones.
- *Metastatic disease:* The most common primary malignancy to affect the GB is melanoma.

### ■ Essential Facts

- This case reviews the imaging similarity between invasive GB carcinoma and XGC, which may be indistinguishable.
- GB carcinoma is:
  - The sixth most common gastrointestinal malignancy, with a 5-year survival rate of < 5% if symptomatic.
  - More common in women older than 60 years of age, American Indians, and Hispanics and associated with porcelain GB, familial polyposis, irritable bowel disease, and gallstones (in 80–100%).
- GB carcinoma imaging may show:
  - Mass within the GB, mass centered in the GB fossa with no identifiable GB (most common), or just wall thickening that is asymmetric or diffuse.
  - Invasion of duodenum, colon, or liver.
  - Periportal, pancreaticoduodenal, hepatic, and celiac lymphadenopathy (common).
  - Peritoneal carcinomatosis and hematogenous metastases.
- XGC is:
  - A chronic inflammatory condition. Like GB carcinoma, it is more common in women 60 to 70 years old with gallstones.
  - Characterized by gray-yellow mural nodules in containing lipid-laden macrophages.
- XGC imaging may show:
  - GB wall thickening with distinctive, hypodense nodules or bands within the GB wall.
  - Multiple masslike loculi with thick septa around pockets of nearly fluid-density material.
  - Invasion of the liver, abdominal wall, or chest wall.
  - Lymphadenopathy (usually less than GB carcinoma).

### ■ Other Imaging Findings

- Ultrasound of GB carcinoma may show wall thickening and intraluminal extension of mural masses, gallstones, porcelain GB, perforation with pericholecystic fluid/stones, and tumor extension into the adjacent hepatic parenchyma.
- Ultrasound of XGC may show characteristic hypoechoic mural nodules or streaks.
- Barium studies of both GB carcinoma and XGC may show invasion and eccentric compression of the adjacent duodenum or colon.

### ✓ Pearls & ✗ Pitfalls

- ✓ XGC is an uncommon type of cholecystitis, and GB carcinoma should be given serious consideration for a thick-walled, multiloculate GB mass.
- ✓ XGC is often associated with GB carcinoma.
- ✓ Acalculous or calculous cholecystitis may result in a contained rupture with an adjacent walled-off abscess. Abdominal wall invasion would be unusual.
- ✗ GB adenocarcinoma may invade the colon, and colon carcinoma may invade the GB. Consider both entities when both organs are involved.

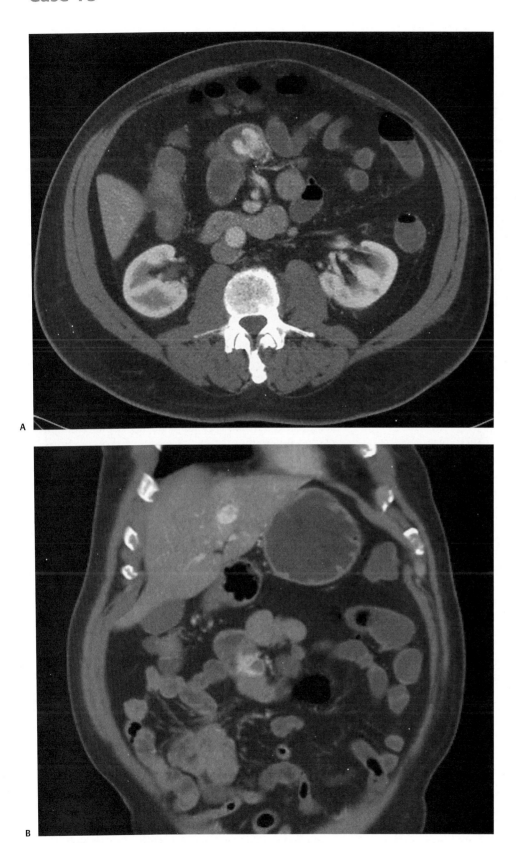

A

B

## Clinical Presentation

A 70-year-old man presents to the gastroenterology clinic with weight loss, nausea, and vomiting.

## ■ Imaging Findings

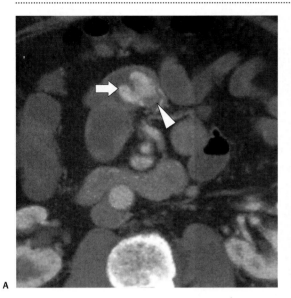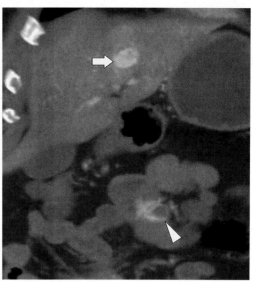

**(A)** Axial contrast-enhanced computed tomography (CT) shows an enhancing polypoid mass (*arrow*) extending into the lumen of the jejunum from a point of attachment to the bowel wall (*arrowhead*). **(B)** Coronal image shows an enhancing mass within the left lobe of the liver (*arrow*) in addition to the jejunal mass (*arrowhead*) with low-density central necrosis.

## ■ Differential Diagnosis

- **Gastrointestinal stromal tumor (GIST):** This is the most likely diagnosis, indicated by a heterogeneous, lobulated polyp with regions of low attenuation after contrast administration.
- *Primary small-bowel adenocarcinoma:* For this diagnosis, appearances range from subtle fold thickening to polyps to infiltrating or ulcerating masses. Although usually found at or near the ampulla, 25% are jejunal.
- *Carcinoid:* Usually in the ileum, carcinoid is often small (< 2 cm), calcified, and associated with a desmoplastic reaction, but it may present as a polyp extending into the lumen without desmoplasia.

## ■ Essential Facts

- GIST is the most common mesenchymal neoplasm, often appearing as an intraluminal polypoid mass with cavitary, cystic, hemorrhagic, and/or exophytic components.
- Location may be intraluminal, submucosal, or subserosal within the stomach (most common), small bowel (second), or any GI location.
- Associated with neurofibromatosis type 1
- CT typically shows a smoothly marginated, enhancing mass with internal, hypoattenuating regions, as in this case.
- CT evidence favoring malignant degeneration of a GIST includes irregular margination with invasion of adjacent organs and metastatic spread, most commonly to liver, as in this case.

- Adenocarcinoma of the small bowel is uncommon, representing less than 2% of GI malignancies. Adenocarcinoma of the jejunum more often presents with stricture from focal, irregularly marginated, annular wall thickening, occasionally with nodal metastases. Associations include celiac and Crohn disease.
- Metastatic disease is the most common small-bowel neoplasm, but it more commonly presents as multiple small-bowel masses, as in malignant melanoma.
- Carcinoid of the jejunum is less commonly an isolated polypoid mass on presentation and often presents with a small mural mass, thickened wall and folds, a retractile desmoplastic reaction, obstruction, prominent nodal metastases, and enhancing liver metastases.
- Lymphoma can appear as a polypoid mass. Usually found in the ileum, lymphoma may be polypoid, but it is more typically associated with mesenteric lymphadenopathy and hypovascular.

## ✓ Pearls & ✗ Pitfalls

- ✓ Polypoid malignancies of the small bowel may be indistinguishable on imaging studies.
- ✗ Do not miss complications of a small-bowel mass, such as intussusception, perforation, ulceration, and obstruction.
- ✗ Intraluminal debris and postinflammatory pseudotumors can mimic polyps. Look for distinguishing neoplastic features, such as enhancement, infiltration, metastasis, and lymphadenopathy.

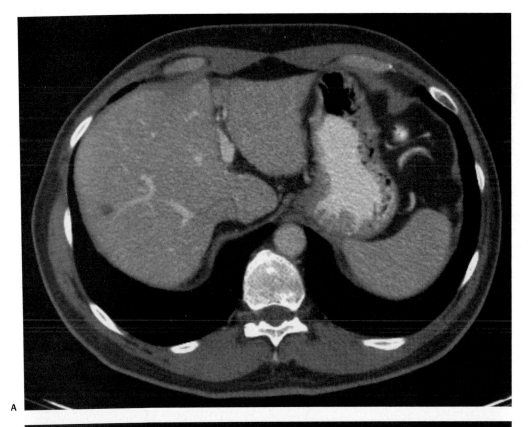

A

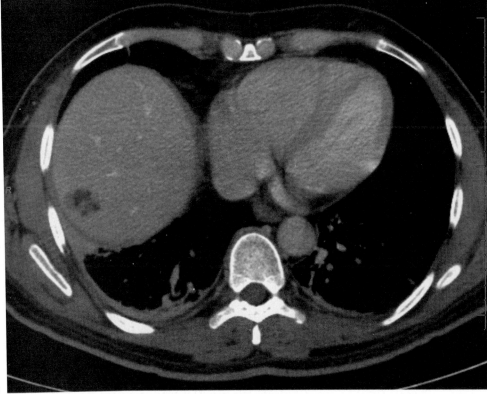

B

## ▪ Clinical Presentation

A 54-year-old woman presents with nausea and weight loss. The second image was obtained 14 months after the first.

## ◼ Imaging Findings

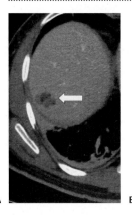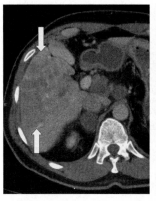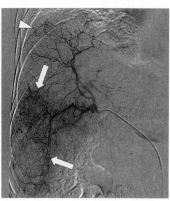

A          B                                                                 C

**(A)** Contrast-enhanced computed tomography (CT) obtained after 14 months shows enlargement and cranial extension of the lesion (*arrow*) in the right lobe of the liver. The lesion is heterogeneous, with foci of fat attenuation as well as slightly hypoattenuating soft tissue. **(B)** More caudal slice shows a large, heterogeneous mass (*arrows*) on the 14-month follow-up study. **(C)** Selected angiogram shows extensive neovascularity in the right lobe (*arrows*), with a focus of neovascularity in the region of the lesion seen on CT (*arrowhead*). This study was obtained in preparation for chemoembolization.

## ◼ Differential Diagnosis

- **Hepatocellular carcinoma (HCC):** This is the principal diagnostic consideration for a growing mass in the liver with patchy macroscopic fat. The rest of the entities on this list are much less common but mentioned for discussion purposes.
- *Liposarcoma (usually metastatic):* This is the second-choice malignancy on the differential for macroscopic fat, but it is very rare in the liver. Rapid growth supports a malignant lesion like liposarcoma or HCC.
- *Angiomyolipomas:* These rarely occur in the liver and typically have a heterogeneous appearance due to enhancing soft-tissue components, ectatic arteries, and foci of macroscopic fat.
- *Teratomas:* These may occur in the liver by metastatic spread, by direct invasion, or as a primary neoplasm. Primary hepatic teratoma is very rare. The combination of soft tissue, fat, and calcification (bone) would be more specific for this entity.

## ◼ Essential Facts

- This case reviews the differential diagnosis for fat-containing liver masses, which may contain microscopic and/or macroscopic fat deposits.
- HCC may contain patchy regions of macroscopic fat in 10 to 35% of cases. HCC is more typically associated with a soft-tissue component that enhances in the early arterial phase, invades vessels, and causes arteriovenous shunting.
- Microscopic interstitial or intracellular fat deposits may be difficult to characterize on CT studies (obtain a chemical shift magnetic resonance imaging [MRI] study). Such masses include focal fatty infiltration, hepatic adenoma, and focal nodular hyperplasia.

- Hepatic adenoma may contain microscopic intracellular fat or focal patches of macroscopic fat that may be quite prominent, with an appearance like that of HCC (< 10% adenomas have fat visible on CT).
- Focal nodular hyperplasia rarely has microscopic intracellular fat and small peripheral patches of macroscopic fat.
- Focal steatosis is microscopic fat occurring in relatively predictable locations: periportal (especially the medial segment of the left lobe), adjacent to the falciform ligament, subcapsular, and adjacent to the gallbladder fossa.
- Other benign masses with macroscopic fat are rare and typically grow more slowly, including angiomyolipoma, myelolipoma, and lipoma.

## ◼ Other Imaging Findings

- MRI is the best modality to identify fat within any tumor, evidenced by increased signal on T1, decreased signal on T2, and signal dropout on out-of-phase gradient-echo images compared with in-phase images (chemical shift).

## ✓ Pearls & ✗ Pitfalls

- ✓ Intrahepatic lipoma is extremely uncommon and typically stable in size, excluding it from the differential diagnosis in this case.
- ✓ Macroscopic fat occurs in both benign and malignant masses and is therefore a nonspecific finding.
- ✓ Look for associated features suspicious for malignancy, such as rapid growth, enhancing soft-tissue components, and vascular invasion.

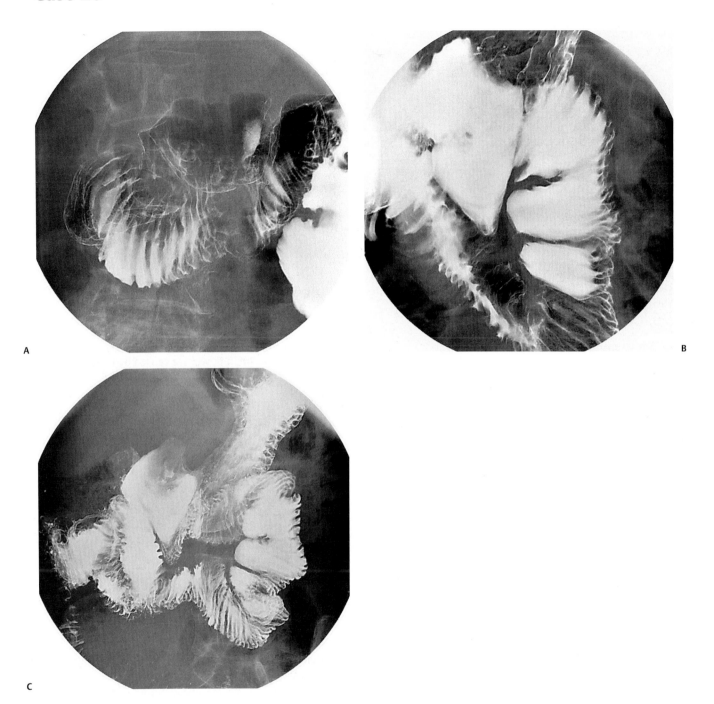

A

B

C

## Clinical Presentation

A 39-year-old woman presents with nausea and abdominal distension.

### ■ Imaging Findings

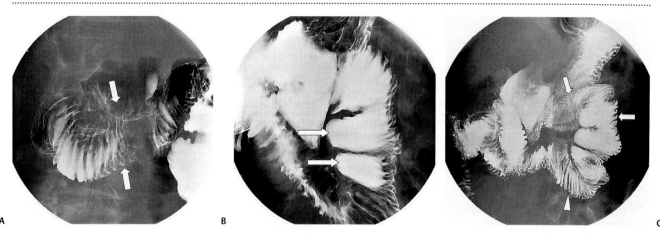

**(A)** Upper gastrointestinal (GI) barium study shows stacks of straight duodenal folds and duodenal dilatation (*arrows*). **(B)** The proximal jejunum is dilated with contrast-filled pseudosacculations (*arrows*). **(C)** Delayed image shows dilatation of the duodenum and jejunum (*arrows*) with stacks of thin, straight folds throughout the jejunum (*arrowhead*).

### ■ Differential Diagnosis

- ***Scleroderma:*** This is the most likely diagnosis, given the stacks of thin, straight duodenal and jejunal folds (hidebound). Note the dilated small bowel, which is most consistent with scleroderma.
- *Small-bowel obstruction:* This may present with dilated loops, but without stacked small-bowel folds.
- *Pseudo-obstruction:* A third option, this may have a similar appearance. It is either idiopathic or caused by systemic diseases with associated neuropathy or myopathy (e.g., dermatomyositis).

### ■ Essential Facts

- Progressive systemic sclerosis (PSS) is thought to be an autoimmune disease. This collagen vascular disease affects small vessels throughout the body and causes fibrosis and collagen deposition.
- PSS most commonly affects the esophagus in the GI tract (80% of GI cases), but the small bowel is commonly involved and heralds more rapid disease progression.
- Hidebound small bowel refers to the finding on barium studies of increased frequency of thin, straight folds (typically jejunal), usually occurring after the onset of skin changes. This finding is also discernable on computed tomography studies with oral contrast.
- Marked small-bowel dilatation (beyond the normal 3-cm diameter) most commonly affects the duodenum, as in this case (termed *megaduodenum*), and less commonly the jejunum.
- No hypersecretion is present with small-bowel scleroderma, unlike in celiac disease.

- Pseudosacculations/pseudodiverticula on the antimesenteric side of the small bowel are caused by foci of smooth muscle atrophy and appear as wide-mouthed, square-topped sacs with diminished folds, as evident in this case.
- Pneumatosis cystoides intestinalis and pneumoperitoneum ("benign" or "balanced") may transiently or continuously occur without symptoms or clinical significance.

### ■ Other Imaging Findings

- Small-bowel series may also show accordion pleating, which is abnormal bowel peristalsis similar to an accordion. Transit time can be markedly prolonged because of abnormal and diminished peristalsis.
- Radiographs may show bilateral basilar interstitial disease, hidebound folds, dilated loops, pneumatosis, and pneumoperitoneum.

### ✓ Pearls & ✗ Pitfalls

- ✓ Intussusception without a lead point can occur with scleroderma.
- ✗ Unnecessary surgery can be avoided by recognizing the benign nature of findings such as small-bowel dilatation and balanced pneumoperitoneum/pneumatosis associated with scleroderma. Correlation with the patient's clinical presentation and history is imperative!
- ✗ Celiac disease causes an increased number of thin folds in the ileum and a decreased number of folds in the jejunum, features distinguishing this entity from PSS.

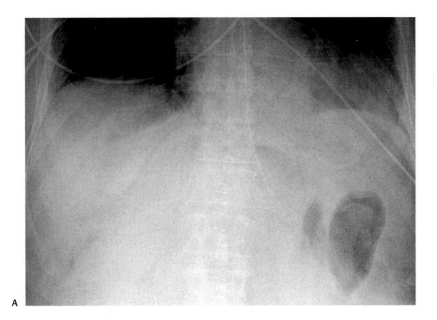

A

**Clinical Presentation**

A 70-year-old man presents with abdominal pain.

**Further Work-up**

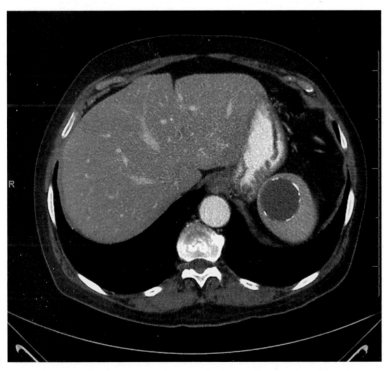

B

### ■ Imaging Findings

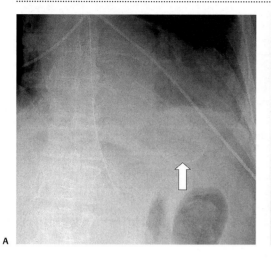 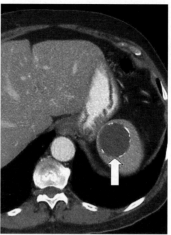

**(A)** Abdominal radiograph shows a curvilinear calcification (*arrow*) projected over the left upper quadrant of the abdomen. **(B)** Infused abdominal computed tomography (CT) shows a round cystic lesion (*arrow*) with a calcified rim.

### ■ Differential Diagnosis

- *Simple splenic cyst:* This is the most likely diagnosis for the CT finding of a fluid-density, nonenhancing, round structure in the spleen. The differential diagnosis for the curvilinear calcification seen on the radiograph is discussed in "Pearls & Pitfalls."
- *Epidermoid cyst:* This may have identical features, although it calcifies less commonly.
- *Echinococcal cyst:* These typically contain debris, cells, and hydatid sand (detached scolices) within the cyst, causing inhomogeneity and increased density.
- *Pancreatic pseudocyst:* This may occur within the splenic parenchyma; however, evidence of associated pancreatitis on imaging studies would be more suggestive of this entity.

### ■ Essential Facts

- Simple splenic cysts are typically the result of past trauma (most commonly), healed abscess, or infarction. They lack an epithelial layer.
  - Infused CT usually shows a single, fluid-density, round, unilocular cyst with an imperceptibly thin wall, often with rim calcifications. Septa are uncommon.
  - Rarely, superinfection, bleeding, or traumatic rupture may occur within a simple splenic cyst.
- Epidermoid cysts are congenital true cysts with an epithelial and mesenchymal lining.
  - Infused CT findings mirror those of simple cysts, although epidermoid cysts have rim calcifications in < 25%.
  - Contents are typically homogeneous, but cholesterol crystals, blood, and fat have been described.
- Echinococcal cysts are the result of *Echinococcus granulosus* infection, and most cases occur within the liver. The spleen is uncommonly affected.

- Infused CT commonly shows internal septa with enhancement of the cyst wall due to a vascular adventitial layer and granulation tissue.
- They expand by budding daughter cysts, which may be seen as peripheral cysts along the rim.
- Eggshell calcifications are common.
- Pancreatic pseudocysts occur within the splenic parenchyma uncommonly, possibly by invasion of splenic parenchyma vessels by pancreatic enzymes.

### ■ Other Imaging Findings

- Ultrasound shows simple splenic cysts to be thin-walled and anechoic, in most cases with posterior acoustic enhancement.
- Rim calcifications may cause shadowing.
- Hemorrhage or superinfection may cause heterogeneity or increased echogenicity.

### ✓ Pearls & ✗ Pitfalls

- ✓ Clinical information is helpful to rule out abscess or infected cyst when the clinician is faced with a splenic fluid collection.
- ✗ Curvilinear calcifications on an abdominal radiograph may be within any projected organ. In this case, consider masses and cysts within the lung, mesentery, omentum, spleen, stomach, small bowel, and colon.
- ✗ Always raise the possibility of a pseudoaneurysm when faced with the radiographic finding of a round or ovoid, peripherally calcified structure.

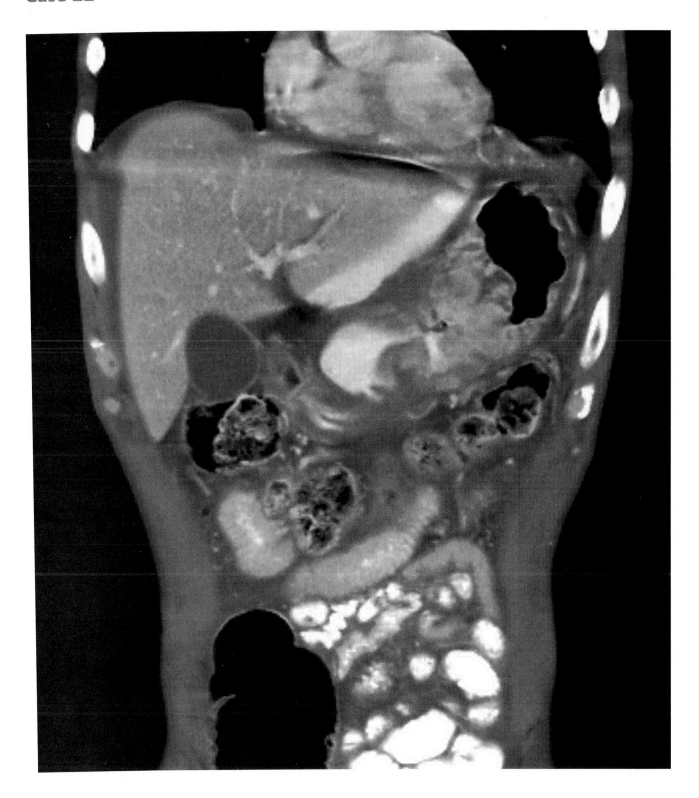

## Clinical Presentation

A 49-year-old man presents with a history of upper gastrointestinal bleeding and new onset of abdominal pain.

### ■ Imaging Findings

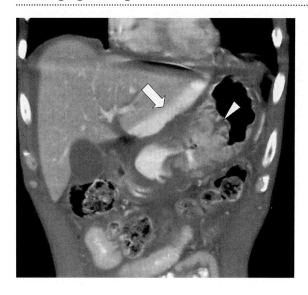

Coronal reformatted contrast-enhanced computed tomography image shows a large, expansile mass (*arrowhead*) within the gastric lumen, adjacent mural thickening, and adjacent extraluminal contrast material (*arrow*). Free air is present below the middiaphragm.

### ■ Differential Diagnosis

- ***Gastric adenocarcinoma with perforation:*** This is the most likely diagnosis, suggested by a fungated, polypoid mass obliterating the gastric lumen and with adjacent mural thickening and extraluminal contrast material.
- *Lymphoma:* This is a possible diagnosis as it may exhibit the same set of possible imaging appearances.
- *Metastasis to the stomach:* This may include melanoma, in addition to breast, lung, pancreatic, and other gastrointestinal primary malignant tumors.

### ■ Essential Facts

- Gastric adenocarcinoma is more common in males, and the gross appearance may be classified as early, infiltrative, or expansile, as in this case.
- Early:
  - Fewer than 25% are diagnosed at this stage.
  - A mucosal or submucosal mass is often picked up incidentally on endoscopic or barium study for symptoms of gastritis.
  - Extension beyond the submucosa and/or associated lymphadenopathy carries a bad prognosis, but the remainder have a 5-year survival rate of 90%.
- Expansile or polypoid:
  - Most commonly villous and well differentiated
  - Occurs equally throughout the stomach
  - Presents with features of this case: a sessile, fungated, often ulcerated, irregularly marginated soft-tissue mass expanding into the lumen
- Infiltrative or scirrhous:
  - Most commonly poorly differentiated, with a dismal prognosis (5-year survival rate < 80%)

- Linitis plastica is progressive invasion of the gastric wall causing marked thickening, a desmoplastic reaction, and loss of peristalsis.
- Ulcerative:
  - Often a feature of expansile type, ulcers are more likely to be malignant on barium studies when the crater appears within the confines of the gastric lumen and is surrounded by focally absent areae gastricae, nodules, or an asymmetric mass.
  - Folds surrounding a malignant ulcer typically terminate short of the ulcer pit.

### ✓ Pearls & ✗ Pitfalls

- ✓ Lymphoma of the stomach is typically non-Hodgkin type and has the same set of possible gross appearances; distinction usually requires endoscopic biopsy.
  - May be nodular, polypoid, ulcerative, or infiltrative
  - As in the small bowel, diffuse infiltration by lymphoma often fails to obstruct the lumen.
  - Perforation is common, particularly during treatment with chemotherapy.
  - Tends to cross the pylorus to involve both the antrum and duodenal bulb
- ✓ Linitis plastica may be caused by gastric adenocarcinoma, lymphoma, tuberculosis, and metastasis from breast and pancreatic carcinoma.
- ✗ Submucosal masses in the stomach may be benign or malignant. Do not forget gastric adenocarcinoma in this differential!

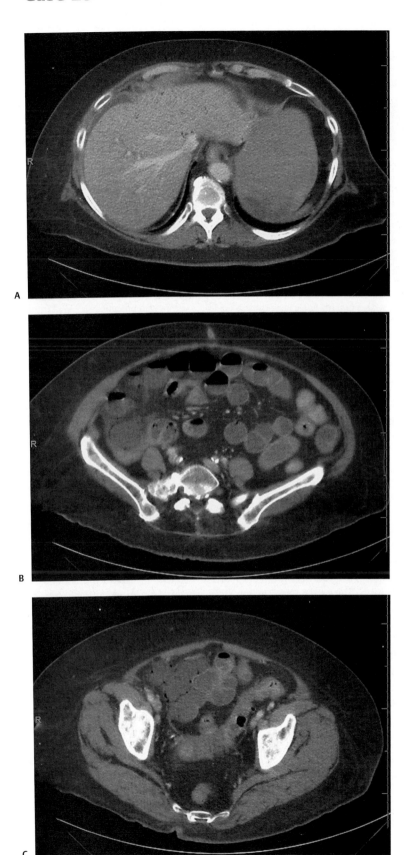

A

B

C

## Clinical Presentation

A 61-year-old woman presents with acute abdominal pain and fever.

## ■ Imaging Findings

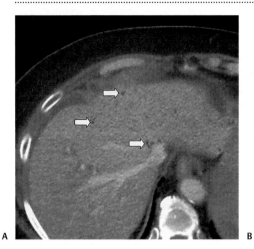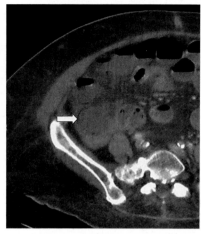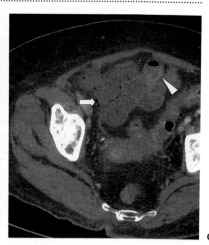

**(A)** Contrast-enhanced abdominal computed tomography (CT) image shows multiple punctate, hypodense foci (*arrows*) in the liver that are difficult to characterize, given their small size, but are suspicious for portal venous gas. **(B)** Pelvic image shows fluid-filled cecum with pneumatosis (*arrow*) and mesenteric fat stranding. **(C)** More caudal image shows multiple loops of distended terminal ileum, some with pneumatosis (*arrow*) and wall thickening (*arrowhead*).

## ■ Differential Diagnosis

- ***Acute mesenteric ischemia (AMI):*** This is the most likely diagnosis, given the findings of portal venous gas, pneumatosis, mesenteric fat stranding, and thickened, distended, fluid-filled terminal ileum and cecum.
- *Infection of the ileum and cecum (*Yersinia *infection, tuberculosis, actinomycosis, and amebiasis):* A consideration, as it can cause pneumatosis, but more bowel wall thickening and exudative fat stranding would be expected.
- *Inflammatory bowel disease:* Crohn disease can involve the ileum and cecum but is less likely in this case, given the limited mural thickening and mesenteric fat infiltration.

## ■ Essential Facts

- AMI describes the acute onset of insufficient oxygen supply to the bowel, usually caused by insufficient blood flow.
- The cause may be occlusive or nonocclusive mesenteric ischemia (NOMI).
- Occlusive AMI is the most common form and may result from arterial embolus, arterial thrombosis, or venous thrombosis. Other possible causes include the acute onset of primary vascular pathology, such as vasculitis, trauma, or dissection.
- Arterial embolus typically involves the distal branches of a mesenteric artery, such as the terminal ileal and ileocolic branches of the superior mesenteric artery, as in this case.
  - Origins of emboli include the heart (myocardial infarction, bacterial endocarditis, atrial fibrillation), aortic plaque or aneurysm, and endovascular procedures.

- Arterial thrombosis typically involves the origin of the affected mesenteric artery, resulting in ischemia to a larger distribution of bowel.
  - Causes of thrombosis include preexisting arterial disease (atherosclerosis, vasculitis, fibromuscular dysplasia) and systemic conditions, such as hypercoagulable states and hypotension.
- Mesenteric venous thrombosis is unlikely in this case because of the limited vascular distribution and the acute onset of symptoms. This entity more typically progresses over weeks and may be idiopathic or secondary to polycythemia, liver or bowel transplant, smoking, hypercoagulable states, and infections.
- NOMI is reduced blood flow to the mesenteric vasculature due to serious illness or pharmacologic effect (vasopressors). Arterial-phase CT shows poor distal mesenteric blood flow and diffuse distribution of ischemic bowel.
  - Causes of NOMI include vasopressors, shock of any etiology, and cardiopulmonary bypass.

## ✓ Pearls & ✗ Pitfalls

- ✓ Pneumatosis and portal venous gas are caused by gas-producing bacteria colonizing necrotic bowel. Other causes include severe infection, radiation therapy, intestinal obstruction, volvulus, and strangulated hernia.
- ✓ Portal venous gas travels to the periphery of the liver, as opposed to biliary gas, which avoids the periphery.
- ✗ AMI can be a life-threatening emergency as bowel necrosis can occur within hours. Early imaging signs should not be missed.

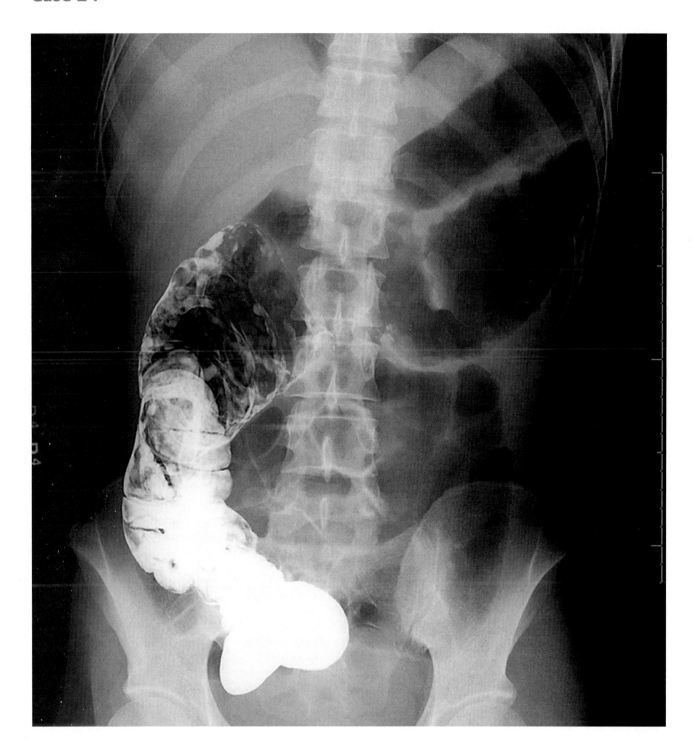

## Clinical Presentation

A 31-year-old man presents with intense abdominal pain. This radiograph was obtained following computed tomography with oral contrast.

### ■ Imaging Findings

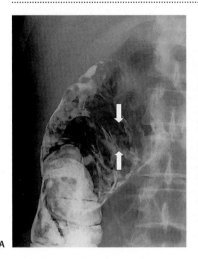 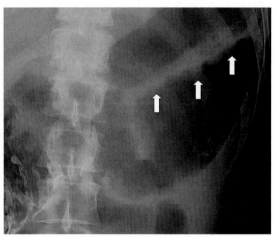

**(A)** Residual barium from a prior computed tomography coats the ascending colon. Innumerable polypoid lesions (*arrows*) are seen throughout the ascending colon, consistent with pseudopolyps, given the appearance of the remainder of the colon (see B). **(B)** The hepatic flexure and transverse colon are markedly dilated, with a thumbprinting pattern along the colonic wall.

### ■ Differential Diagnosis

- ***Toxic megacolon due to ulcerative colitis (UC):*** This is the most likely diagnosis, given the combination of pseudopolyps, marked colonic dilatation, and thumbprinting. UC is mentioned first because it is the most frequent cause of toxic megacolon.
- *Ischemic colitis:* This also causes thumbprinting, pseudopolyps, and toxic megacolon.
- *Pseudomembranous colitis:* This can cause toxic megacolon. A history of broad-spectrum antibiotic use, sepsis, mesenteric ischemia, or neoplasm would be supportive.

### ■ Essential Facts

- UC is an inflammatory bowel disease of unknown etiology that is usually limited to the mucosa, as opposed to Crohn disease, which is usually transmural.
- Toxic megacolon is the most common cause of death due to UC and occurs in up to 10% of patients with UC.
  - Clinical diagnosis is the key and is based on an increased sedimentation rate, fever, leukocytosis, and anemia. The anemia is caused by marked bloody diarrhea.
  - Fulminant colitis is associated with marked colonic dilatation (≥ 10 cm in the cecum, ≥ 6 cm elsewhere) or a rapidly increasing diameter on radiographs with a loss of haustral folds.
  - Transmural involvement of the colon manifests as deeper extension of normally shallow ulcerations and inflammation, extending to the serosa. It may involve the pericolonic fat and peritoneum with or without frank colonic perforation.
  - Pseudopolyps represent remnant patches of mucosa surrounded by severely ulcerated and denuded bowel wall.

- Pneumatosis and peritonitis may result.
- Pneumoperitoneum may be seen in the event of frank rupture.

### ■ Other Imaging Findings

- Barium enema:
  - Is absolutely contraindicated when toxic megacolon is suspected because of the high risk for rupture.
  - May be an exacerbating factor leading to toxic megacolon in patients with UC.

### ✓ Pearls & ✗ Pitfalls

- ✓ Tuberculosis (TB) affects the ileum and cecum and sometimes involves the ascending colon, but the extent of involvement in this case makes TB unlikely. In the hypertrophic (vs. ulcerative) form, transmural involvement can cause thumbprinting, pseudopolyps, mural thickening, and toxic megacolon. Coned cecum is more classic.
- ✓ Toxic megacolon can occur in association with Crohn disease, TB colitis, and amebiasis.
- ✓ Infectious forms of colitis, such as amebiasis and strongyloidiasis, can cause pseudopolyps.
- ✗ Loss of the haustral folds does not indicate toxic megacolon. This finding occurs with chronic UC.
- ✗ Lack of colonic dilatation does not rule out toxic megacolon. An appropriate clinical presentation in a patient who has UC, coupled with suspect features such as thumbprinting, should raise suspicion for this entity.

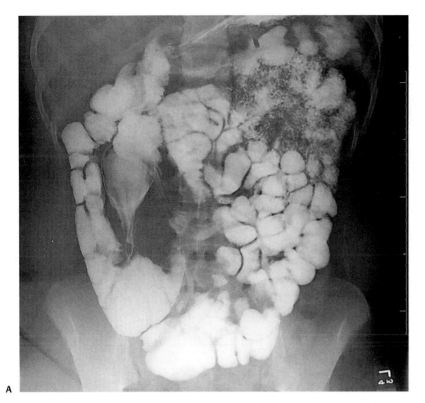

A

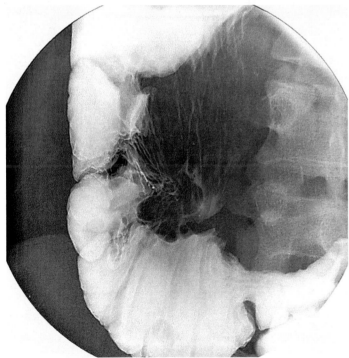

B

## ▇ Clinical Presentation

An 18-year-old woman presents with intermittent right lower quadrant pain.

### ■ Imaging Findings

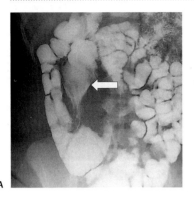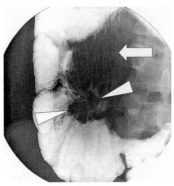

A                                                                                                          B

**(A)** Small-bowel follow-through shows a dilated, patulous terminal ileum (*arrow*) with diffuse effacement of the mucosal folds. Dilution of barium in the distal small bowel suggests a pattern of malabsorption. **(B)** Compression view with the cecum maximally distended shows an enlarged, nodular ileocecal valve (*arrowheads*) surrounded by a tethered appearance on the mesenteric side of the surrounding colon. The *arrow* indicates residual barium within the patulous terminal ileum.

### ■ Differential Diagnosis

- *Crohn disease:* Crohn disease is a common cause of nodular thickening of the ileocecal valve and pericecal inflammation, causing deformity related to fibrotic tethering. Dilatation of the terminal ileum is a feature less common than stricture formation with chronic Crohn disease, but prestenotic dilatation can occur because of backwash ileitis or a focal stricture at or near the ileocecal valve.
- *Ulcerative colitis:* This can cause ileocecal valve deformity and an effaced terminal ileum due to backwash ileitis.
- *Infection (tuberculosis):* This may mimic the features of Crohn disease in the terminal ileum and cecum, including ileocecal valve enlargement and deformity.
- *Carcinoid:* This has a predilection for the terminal ileum and can involve the ileocecal valve or prolapse into the cecum, with associated fibrotic tethering due to desmoplastic reaction.

### ■ Essential Facts

- This case reviews the differential diagnosis for enlargement and deformity of the ileocecal valve on barium studies. Characterize the ileocecal valve by size, shape, and any associated abnormalities of the terminal ileum or cecum, as in this case.
- The ileocecal valve should be evaluated during maximal cecal distension and is typically < 4 cm in diameter on barium studies.
- The ileocecal valve can appear polypoid to somewhat nodular, usually on the medial cecum along the first haustral fold.
- Enlargement without deformity of the adjacent bowel may indicate a mass (see "Pearls & Pitfalls").
- Deformity of the valve can occur with any local neoplasm, infection, inflammation, or intussusception.

### ■ Other Imaging Findings

- Barium studies of an abnormal ileocecal valve may show incompetence of the valve during double-contrast studies; an irregular, lobulated contour; a carpetlike appearance (of villous adenoma); and abnormal contour of the adjacent cecal wall or haustral fold.

### ✓ Pearls & ✗ Pitfalls

- ✓ Lipomatous infiltration is the most common cause of ileocecal valve enlargement and is non-neoplastic fat deposition that is more symmetric than lipoma.
- ✓ Lipoma is the most common benign neoplasm of the ileocecal valve. This lesion is distinguished by its variable shape, nodular appearance, and compressibility on barium studies.
- ✓ Other benign lesions of the ileocecal valve include polypoid lesions, such as adenomas and lipomas, and nodular thickening from inflammatory bowel disease or infectious colitis. Consider *Yersinia* infection, tuberculosis, and amebiasis.
- ✓ Malignant lesions affecting the ileocecal valve include adenocarcinoma and lymphoma.
- ✓ Terminal ileum malignancies, such as lymphoma or carcinoid, can prolapse into the cecum and present as an enlarged ileocecal valve.
- ✗ Partial prolapse of the ileum into the cecum is normal but accentuated by incomplete cecal distension; it should not be confused with ileocecal valve enlargement or ileocecal intussusception.

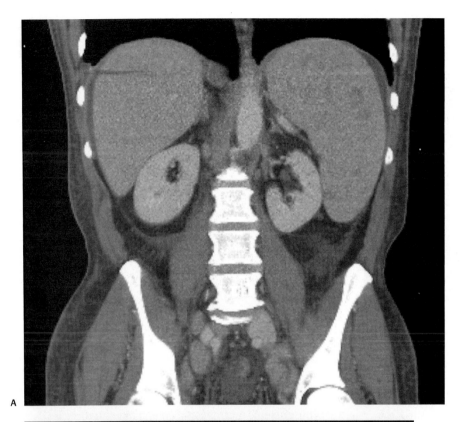

A

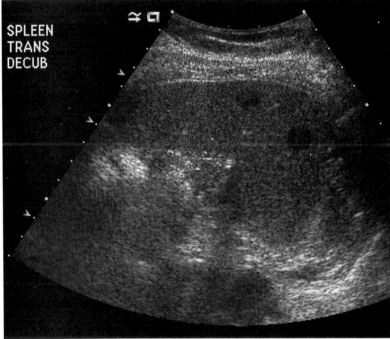

B

## ▪ Clinical Presentation

.....................................................................................................................................................

A 57-year-old man presents with nausea, weight loss, and thrombocytopenia. Ignore the linear artifact in the dome of the liver.

### ■ Imaging Findings

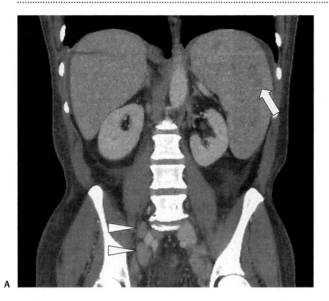
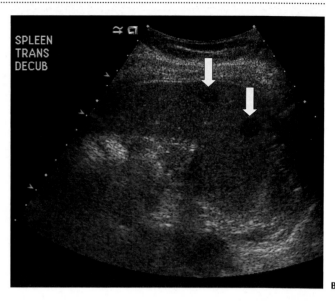

**(A)** Coronal reformatted infused computed tomography (CT) shows splenomegaly with heterogeneous mottling and focal, hypodense lesions (*arrow*). The *arrowheads* indicate enlarged iliac chain lymph nodes. **(B)** Ultrasound shows round, hypoechoic lesions (*arrows*) in the spleen and coarse echotexture.

### ■ Differential Diagnosis

- *Lymphoma:* This is the most common neoplasm of the spleen that appears both hypoechoic and hypodense, as in this case. The enlarged iliac chain nodes are supportive.
- *Infection by* Candida, *tuberculosis, and bacterial infection:* Infection can cause diffuse infiltration as well as focal, hypodense lesions of variable echogenicity. Multiple abscesses can result from septic emboli, usually of cardiac origin.
- *Metastases to the spleen:* These are uncommon and include melanoma as well as breast and lung primaries. These lesions are often echogenic and enhance on infused CT, unlike lymphoma (and this case).

### ■ Essential Facts

- Lymphoma is the most common malignancy involving the spleen, usually occurring in the setting of diffuse abdominal and pelvic disease.
- Focal splenic lesions can be seen in both Hodgkin and non-Hodgkin lymphoma.
- Gastrointestinal lymphoma most commonly involves the stomach and (less commonly) the small bowel.
- Complications include splenic rupture and hemorrhage. However, most patients experience no symptoms related to splenic involvement.

### ■ Other Imaging Findings

- Diffuse splenic mottling and enlargement in this case suggest low-grade lymphomatous infiltration.
- Characteristically hypoechoic and hypodense nodules in this case suggest higher-grade lymphoma.
- Splenic and hepatic lesions in combination are highly suggestive of lymphoma. The liver is typically not involved without splenic involvement.
- Bulky adenopathy adjacent to the spleen or in distant locations is highly suggestive of lymphoma. Look for a mass of coalesced adenopathy in the mesentery.

### ✓ Pearls & ✗ Pitfalls

- ✓ Splenomegaly is usually present when the spleen exceeds 12 cm from pole to pole and 7 cm in width.
- ✓ Normal spleen on imaging studies:
  - CT: hypodense to normal liver
  - Ultrasound: isoechoic to slightly hyperechoic to liver and left kidney

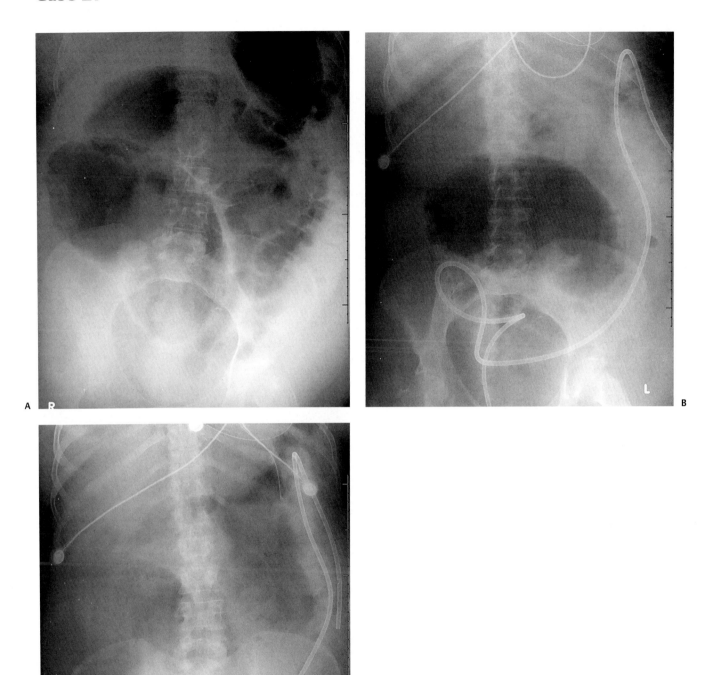

## Clinical Presentation

A 67-year-old woman presents with abdominal distension and pain. Three serial radiographs were obtained over 2 days.

■ **Imaging Findings**

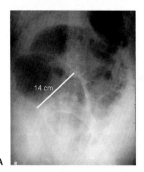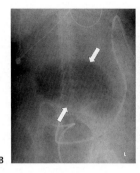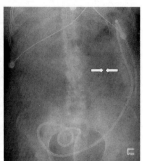

**(A)** Frontal abdominal radiograph shows a dilated loop of bowel in the right lower quadrant measuring 14 cm in diameter. **(B)** After placement of a tube through the rectum for decompression, the entire colon decompressed except for this dilated loop (*arrows*). **(C)** Follow-up radiograph shows decompression of the dilated loop with massive intra-abdominal free air, as evidenced by the Rigler sign (*arrows*).

■ **Differential Diagnosis**

• **_Cecal volvulus with rupture:_** This is the most likely diagnosis, indicated by the dilated, air-filled proximal colon (> 10 cm), by failure to evacuate this segment with a rectal drain despite decompression of the transverse and distal colon, as well as by the ultimate finding of pneumoperitoneum. Cecal volvulus more typically presents as a midline or left upper quadrant dilated loop on radiographs, although the appearance can vary based on the length of the mesentery and mobility of the cecum.
• *Cecal bascule:* This is less prone to rupture but can present with this imaging appearance.
• *Colon carcinoma:* This (or other obstructing mass) may cause progressive dilation proximal to the point of obstruction, but rapid progression is somewhat atypical. Superimposed volvulus or cecal-cecal intussusception can progress more rapidly.

■ **Essential Facts**

• Two key points in this case are the recognition of cecal obstruction and the diagnosis of the life-threatening complication of perforation. The radiographic signs of abdominal free air should be mastered and are outlined below.
• The increased mobility of the ascending and sigmoid colon caused by a longer mesentery predisposes these portions of the large bowel to obstruction—in the cecum less commonly than sigmoid.
• Two types of positional cecal obstruction:
  • Axial cecal volvulus is rotation of the right colon/small bowel around the mesentery (90% of cases of positional cecal obstruction). Supine radiographs usually show a dilated midline loop, more often in the midabdomen to left upper quadrant.
  • Cecal bascule is cranial folding of the cecum (10% of cases of positional cecal obstruction). Radiographs show a gas collection separated from the ascending colon by a transverse fold.

• Causes: cecal volvulus may be iatrogenic (after surgery, colonoscopy) or associated with adhesions, an atonic colon, pregnancy, and neoplasms.
• Presentation is pain, distension, and obstipation.
• Radiographic signs of pneumoperitoneum are the following:
  • Rigler sign: gas on both sides of bowel wall
  • Triangle sign: gas in a triangular space between juxtaposed bowel loops
  • Double-wall sign: double-contrast appearance of bowel loops due to gas inside and out
  • Falciform ligament, umbilical ligament (inverted "V"), ligamentum teres, or urachus signs: gas on both sides of these ligaments

■ **Other Imaging Findings**

• Computed tomography with oral and rectal contrast:
  • Whirl sign is pathognomonic for volvulus but not cecal bascule and is indicative of mesenteric vessels twisted around the axis of the ileocolic artery.
  • Ischemic change is indicated by mural thickening, mesenteric edema, portal venous gas, or pneumatosis.
• Single-contrast barium enema:
  • Barium enema may reduce volvulus or bascule, but instill contrast slowly to avoid perforation.
  • Beak sign on barium studies is a tapered colonic obstruction, often ending with a twist, and indicates axial cecal volvulus, not cecal bascule.
  • Ischemic change: thumbprinting, ulceration

✓ **Pearls & ✗ Pitfalls**

✓ Cecum > 10 cm heralds rupture.
✓ The cecum often dilates out of proportion to the remainder of the colon, even in cases of distal obstruction.

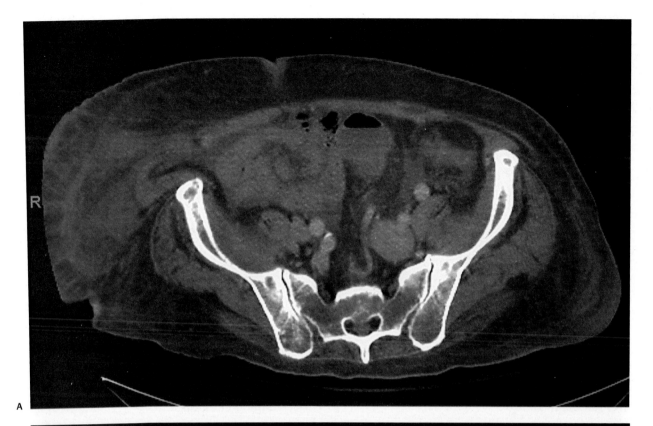

A

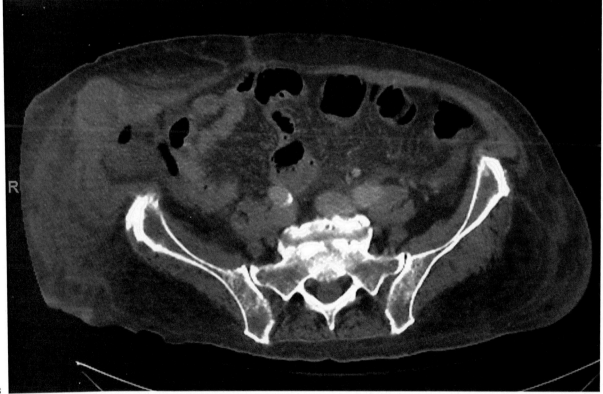

B

## ■ Clinical Presentation

A 65-year-old man presents with a palpable mass in the right lower quadrant of the abdomen.

### ■ Imaging Findings

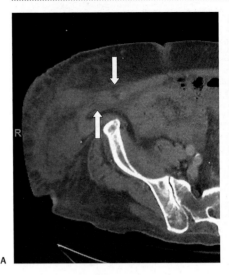 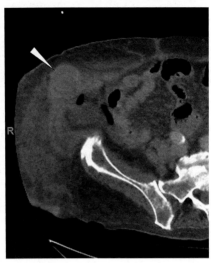

A                                                                                                B

**(A)** Linear strands of soft tissue suggestive of mesenteric blood vessels cross a defect in the abdominal wall just anterior to the iliac spine, between the fibers of the rectus abdominis muscle and the fibers of the transversalis abdominis and internal oblique muscles (*arrows*). **(B)** A pocket of gas lies just at the abdominal wall defect within the abdomen, and a thick-walled, fluid-filled structure (*arrowhead*) lies peripheral to this gas pocket within the abdominal wall.

### ■ Differential Diagnosis

- ***Spigelian hernia (SH):**** This is the most likely diagnosis, given the apparent passage of abdominal contents lateral to the rectus abdominis muscle through the transversalis abdominis and internal oblique muscles.
- *Abdominal wall abscess:* A less likely explanation, given the abdominal wall defect. However, this entity can appear as a fluid-filled, walled-off structure surrounded by edematous fat, as in this case. Origins may include appendicitis and diverticulitis.
- *Primary or metastatic tumor of the abdominal wall:* This may appear as a fluid-filled mass with surrounding fat infiltration. The finding in this case is more likely to be a "pseudotumor," which is a fluid-filled, strangulated bowel with the appearance of a tumor.

### ■ Essential Facts

- SHs are congenital ventral abdominal wall hernias.
- SHs occur at the linea semilunaris, a line extending craniad from the symphysis pubis lateral to the rectus abdominis muscle.
- Contents of SHs pass between the rectus and the combination of the transversalis and internal oblique muscles and are contained by an overlying, intact external oblique muscle, which can be difficult to discern on computed tomography (CT).
- SHs are ventral abdominal hernias, as are incisional hernias from prior abdominal surgery and umbilical hernias.
- SHs are external hernias, as are femoral, inguinal, sciatic notch, and obturator hernias. External hernias exit the abdominal cavity.

### ■ Other Imaging Findings

- Ultrasound is often helpful in cases of suspected external hernia. The identification of peristaltic bowel within a palpable mass is diagnostic.

### ✓ Pearls & ✗ Pitfalls

- ✓ Closed-loop obstruction describes complete obstruction of both ends of a segment of bowel, as in this case. The segment is at risk for necrosis and is often dilated, thick-walled, and fluid-filled.
- ✓ Pseudotumor on CT or radiograph is a segment of obstructed, fluid-filled bowel with the appearance of a tumor, as in this case. This appearance places the patient at high risk for necrosis.
- ✓ Incisional hernias are postsurgical, external abdominal wall hernias occurring at this and other abdominal locations. They are not SHs because they are iatrogenic, not congenital.
- ✓ Umbilical hernias occur through a weakness in the anterior abdominal wall in a periumbilical location.
- ✗ Incarcerated hernias cannot be reduced and may lead to strangulation of bowel.
- ✗ Strangulation of herniated bowel is a mechanical obstruction with interrupted blood flow, placing the patient at risk for necrosis. Imaging findings include bowel wall thickening, distension of the bowel lumen by fluid, and adjacent fat stranding from edema or exudate.
- ✗ Necrosis is indicated by pneumatosis, pneumoperitoneum from perforation, and portal or mesenteric venous gas.

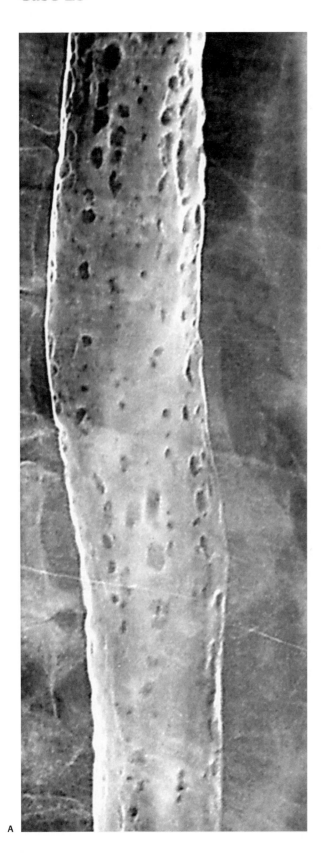

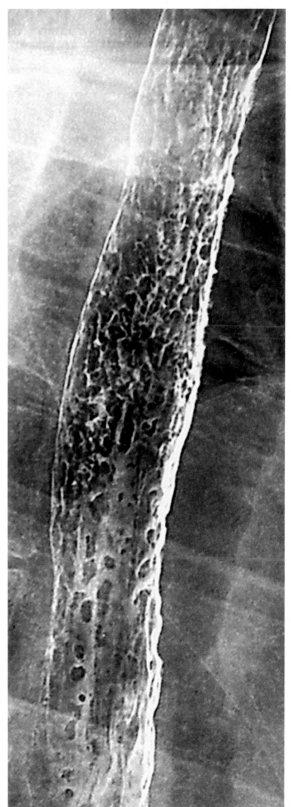

A

B

## Clinical Presentation

An 85-year-old man who has myelodysplastic syndrome and is on prednisone presents with chest pain.

## ■ Imaging Findings

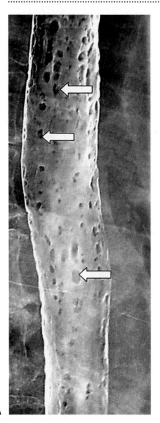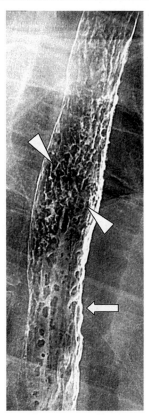

A
B

**(A)** Single-contrast barium study shows innumerable irregularly marginated mucosal nodules (*arrows*) that are linearly arranged. **(B)** Double-contrast study shows irregular mucosal contour (*arrow*) and confluent, shaggy, erosive changes throughout the esophagus (*arrowheads*).

## ■ Differential Diagnosis

- **Candida *esophagitis:*** This is the most likely diagnosis, given the diffuse, shaggy mucosal abnormalities and the clinical history of an elderly patient with a chronic disease being treated with steroids.
- *Viral esophagitis:* In its advanced form, this can be indistinguishable from *Candida* esophagitis.
- *Corrosive esophagitis:* This may have this appearance in the acute stage following ingestion.

## ■ Essential Facts

- *Candida* esophagitis occurs in individuals with chronic debilitating disease, immune compromise, diabetes, and primary or secondary esophageal motility disorders.
- This entity may affect the entire esophagus in some cases but is most common in the distal half.
- Clinical presentation is odynophagia and dysphagia, but immunocompromised patients may present with disseminated infection, multiple-organ involvement, and hemodynamic compromise.
- Barium study findings:
  - Nodularity results from colonies of *Candida* on eroding, edematous esophageal mucosa.

- Shaggy mucosal contour results from continued mucosal erosion coupled with the coalescence of nodules and plaques as *Candida* colonies enlarge.
- Strictures may be a delayed complication of any form of esophagitis.

## ✓ Pearls & ✗ Pitfalls

- ✓ Fine nodularity (1–2 mm) has a broad differential that includes most forms of esophagitis.
- ✓ Consider infectious, pharmacologic, corrosive, and reflux esophagitis.
- ✓ Larger nodules (3–4 mm) may be caused by benign or malignant conditions in addition to opportunistic infections. Benign causes include glycogen acanthosis and epidermolysis bullosa.
- ✓ Malignant nodularity is caused by superficially spreading esophageal carcinoma.
- ✓ Viral esophagitis is indistinguishable from *Candida* esophagitis in its advanced stages but is more distinguishable in the early stages by characteristic ulcerations: broad-based in cytomegalovirus infection and focal in herpes simplex type 1 (occasionally diamond-shaped).

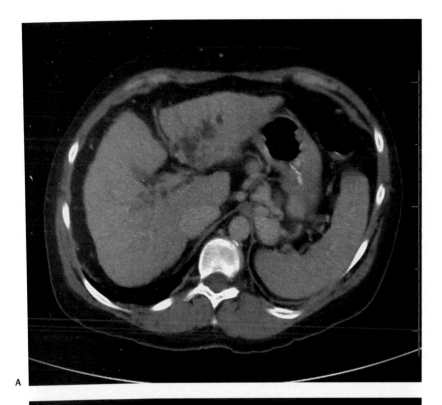

A

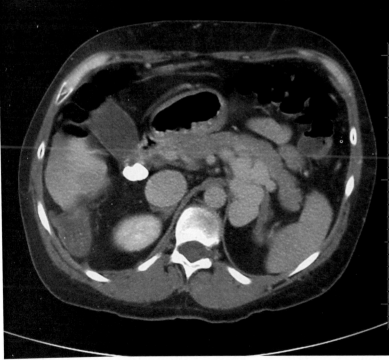

B

## ■ Clinical Presentation

A 47-year-old woman with a history of cirrhosis presents with jaundice, acute right upper quadrant abdominal pain, and fever.

### ■ Imaging Findings

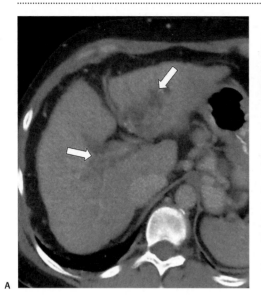
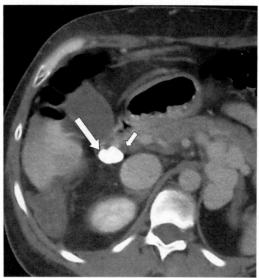

A                                                                                          B

**(A)** Contrast-enhanced computed tomography shows bilateral intrahepatic biliary dilatation (*arrows*) and a shrunken liver, consistent with the provided history of cirrhosis. **(B)** A more caudal image shows a calcified stone (*large arrow*) within the expected location of the gallbladder neck or cystic duct. This stone abuts the common bile duct (CBD; *small arrow*). The incidental finding of a hypodense lesion in the visualized portion of the right lobe of the liver was determined to be hepatoma.

### ■ Differential Diagnosis

- ***Mirizzi syndrome and a hepatoma:*** Mirizzi syndrome is indicated by bilateral intrahepatic biliary dilatation, jaundice with acute right upper quadrant pain, and a large cystic duct stone abutting a CBD of normal caliber. The large stone in this case is strongly indicative of Mirizzi syndrome, but the following entities are mentioned for completeness.
- *Cholangiocarcinoma:* This can cause bilateral duct dilatation despite a normal-caliber CBD.
- *Benign biliary stricture:* Prior infection, surgery, or sclerosing cholangitis can result in bilateral biliary dilatation.

### ■ Essential Facts

- The symptoms and imaging findings in this case raise the possibility of acute biliary obstruction coupled with acute cholecystitis; this combination is most commonly caused by either Mirizzi syndrome or a CBD stone.
- Gallstones obstructing the gallbladder neck or cystic duct typically result in cholecystitis. The biliary tree is not dilated unless a gallstone lodges in the CBD or the patient develops Mirizzi syndrome.
- Mirizzi syndrome occurs when a gallstone lodges in the neck of the gallbladder or cystic duct, resulting in compression of the CBD.

- In Mirizzi syndrome, the CBD diameter is normal at or below the level of the cystic duct, ruling out a stone obstructing the distal CBD as a cause of intrahepatic biliary dilatation.
- Supportive imaging evidence for cholecystitis has not yet developed in this case and would include gallbladder wall thickening, gallbladder distension, pericholecystic fluid, and/or fat stranding.

### ■ Other Imaging Findings

- Ultrasound findings consistent with acute cholecystitis coupled with intrahepatic biliary dilatation should raise suspicion for Mirizzi syndrome.

### ✓ Pearls & ✗ Pitfalls

- ✓ Gallbladder carcinoma or cholangiocarcinoma can cause simultaneous obstruction of the gallbladder and CBD, mimicking Mirizzi syndrome.
- ✓ In any patient with cirrhosis, do not miss a life-threatening hepatoma!

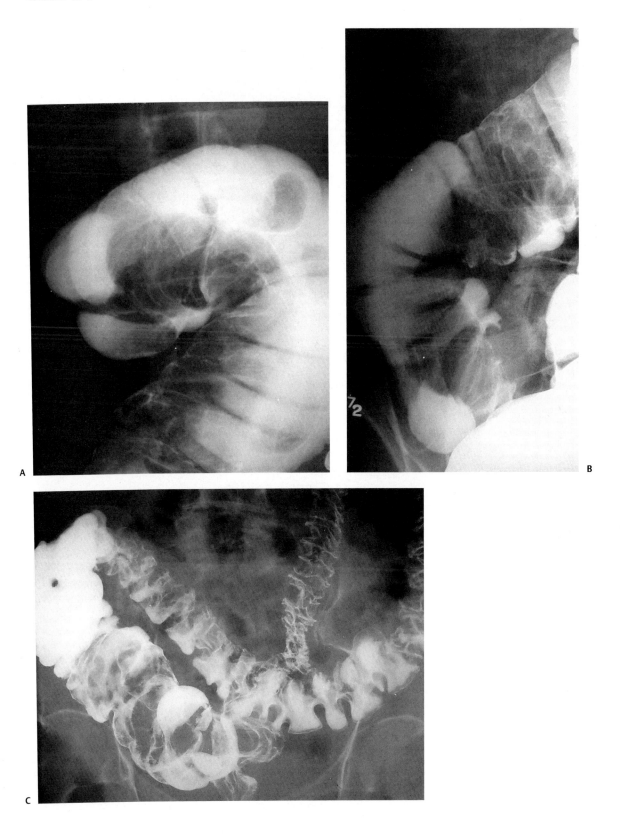

## Clinical Presentation

A 60-year-old man presents to the emergency department with the recent onset of progressive, severe abdominal pain.

## ■ Imaging Findings

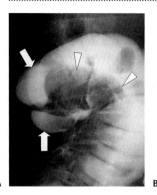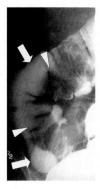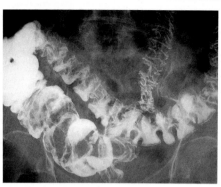

**(A)** Barium enema shows abrupt obstruction of the barium column (*arrows*). A long filling defect (*arrowheads*) invaginates into the lumen. **(B)** Continued filling pushes the barium column to the level of the cecum (*arrows*). The long filling defect (*arrowheads*) appears to originate from the ileocecal level. **(C)** Postevacuation image shows contrast throughout the colon and entering the distal small bowel.

## ■ Differential Diagnosis

- ***Intussusception with a lead point:*** This is the most likely diagnosis, given the verification of intussusception by successful reduction barium enema and considering the age of the patient. This patient should undergo colonoscopy to determine the type of lead point.
- *Intussusception without a lead point:* Intussusception sans a lead point is much less common in adult patients.

## ■ Essential Facts

- Intussusception occurs when peristasis causes a segment of bowel (intussusceptum) to prolapse into an adjacent segment (intussuscipiens).
- Incidence is < 1% of bowel obstructions; it occurs at any age, but only 5% occur in adults.
- Clinical presentation is usually recurrent colicky pain or persistent abdominal pain, nausea, and vomiting.
- The cause may be idiopathic. Both benign and malignant intussusceptions may occur with or without a causative lead point. More than 80% of adult cases are caused by a tumor as the lead point.
- Common locations are colocolic, ileocecal, ileocolic, enterocolic, and points of bowel fixation (e.g., ileocecal region, adhesions).
- Large-bowel intussusceptions more commonly occur with a lead point (> 50%).
- Small-bowel intussusceptions more commonly occur without a lead point; when a lead point is present, the cause is usually benign.
  - Causes of cases without a lead point include celiac disease and Crohn disease.
  - Causes of cases with a lead point include Meckel diverticulum and neoplasms such as metastatic melanoma, lymphoma, primary adenocarcinoma, and benign polyps.
- Imaging studies may detect and characterize a lead structure, intraluminal mesenteric fat and vasculature, and thickened bowel wall.

## ■ Other Imaging Findings

- Computed tomography (CT) of transient intussusception without a lead point shows a sausage-shaped or target-like intraluminal mass.
- The classic CT finding of three layers of bowel wall may be present. If a lead point is present, this classic finding may transition to a simple intraluminal mass, although this distinction is often difficult.

## ✓ Pearls & ✗ Pitfalls

- ✓ Intraluminal polypoid masses are the most likely to cause intussusception as they are advanced forward by peristalsis.
- ✗ Increased use of CT has resulted in the increased detection of transient (often asymptomatic) intussusception without a lead point, likely with no clinical significance. The need for follow-up of such cases is a topic of debate.
- ✗ On barium studies, intraluminal masses, diverticula, and debris, as well as intramural hematomas, can mimic intussusception.
- ✗ Reduction of an intussusception should be avoided in patients with frank ischemic bowel or with strong evidence of a malignant tumor as a lead point.
- ✗ Thickened, edematous bowel within an intussusceptum can mimic a lead point mass by effacing intussuscepted mesenteric fat and vessels.

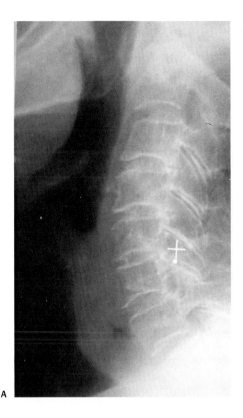

A

## Clinical Presentation

A 56-year-old woman presents with dysphagia.

## Further Work-up

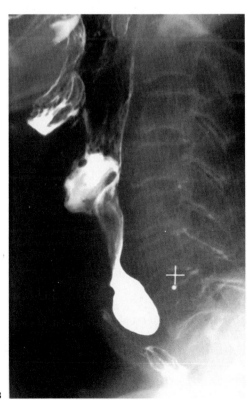

B

### ■ Imaging Findings

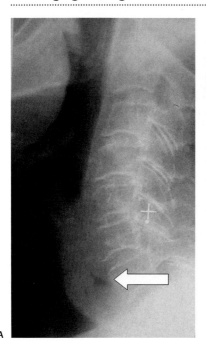
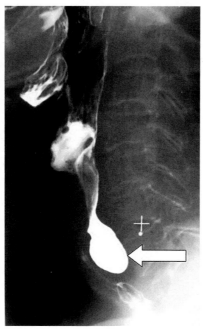

A                                                                                                                                B

**(A)** Lateral radiograph of the neck shows widening of the retrotracheal soft-tissue space and a small focus of gas (*arrow*). **(B)** Lateral radiograph during a barium swallow shows retention of barium in a saccular structure (*arrow*) within the retrotracheal soft tissues. This structure communicates with the pharyngoesophageal junction.

### ■ Differential Diagnosis

- ***Zenker diverticulum (ZD):*** ZD is the most likely diagnosis, given the absence of clinical information suggesting infection or foreign body. A chronic history of bad breath and the periodic regurgitation of foul-smelling food would further support this diagnosis. The barium study findings are pathognomonic for ZD. This differential list is for the radiographic findings.
- *Pharyngeal perforation:* This could present as retropharyngeal gas and barium, but there is no history of an acute episode of foreign body penetration.
- *Retrotracheal abscess:* This third option is more likely if further clinical information indicated the recent onset of fever and leukocytosis.

### ■ Essential Facts

- Retropharyngeal gas is a nonspecific finding that must be tied to the clinical presentation before rank ordering the differential diagnosis. The barium study is pathognomonic for ZD.
- ZD is herniation of the mucosa and submucosa at the cricopharyngeus muscle in the midline of the Killian dehiscence (between oblique and transverse fibers). This level is the pharyngoesophageal junction, typically at C5-C6. ZD is a pulsion diverticulum.
- The cause is unknown, but postulated mechanisms include the following:
  - Abnormal motility at the level of the cricopharyngeus muscle, causing increased pressure
  - Repeated muscular contraction to clear gastroesophageal reflux

- Clinical presentation is typically bad breath, regurgitation of foul-smelling food after meals and at night, and dysphagia. More serious complications include aspiration pneumonia and esophageal obstruction due to extrinsic compression.
- Barium swallow in the lateral projection is the best test and shows a retrotracheal sac communicating with the pharyngoesophageal junction via a narrow neck, sometimes causing extrinsic compression of the proximal esophagus.

### ✓ Pearls & ✗ Pitfalls

- ✓ Killian-Jamieson diverticula are smaller pulsion diverticula occurring laterally or anterolaterally just below the transverse portion of the cricopharyngeus muscle. They are less likely to retain contents than ZD.
- ✓ Traction diverticula may occur throughout the length of the esophagus and typically result from fibrosis due to previous infection, inflammation, or surgery; they are commonly midthoracic diverticula at the level of prior inflammation of hilar and mediastinal adenopathy. Traction diverticula have a variety of shapes and sizes.
- ✓ Pulsion diverticula are typically related to increased intraluminal pressure at points of weakness or dysmotility and include ZD, Killian-Jamieson diverticula, and epiphrenic diverticula. They tend to be saccular.
- ✗ Mimics of diverticula include large ulcerations related to infection or neoplasm, and esophageal rupture. The appearance and clinical history should distinguish these entities from diverticula.

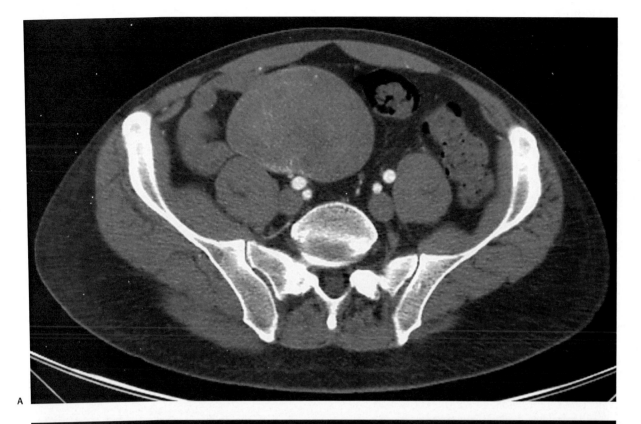

A

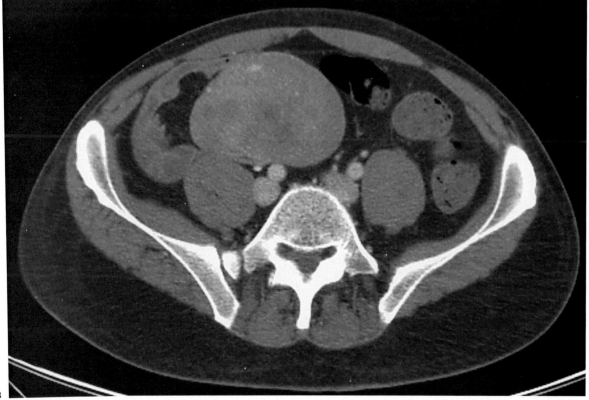

B

## ■ Clinical Presentation

A 52-year-old man with an abdominal mass palpated during a routine physical examination.

## ■ Imaging Findings

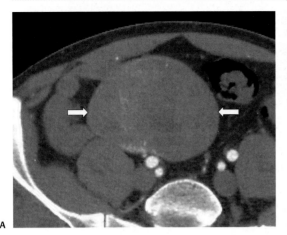 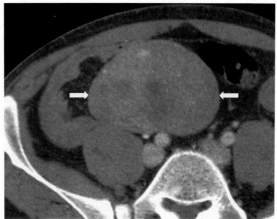

A                                                                      B

**(A)** Arterial-phase contrast-enhanced computed tomography (CT) shows a large, well-circumscribed, homogeneous mass (*arrows*) in the pelvic mesentery. **(B)** Venous-phase image shows heterogeneous enhancement of this mass (*arrows*).

## ■ Differential Diagnosis

- **Gastrointestinal stromal tumor (GIST):** GIST is the first choice for a smoothly marginated mass in the mesentery with heterogeneous enhancement.
- *Desmoid tumor (mesenteric fibromatosis):* This entity may be large and well-circumscribed with heterogeneous or homogeneous enhancement. It is most common in younger women (20–40 years of age). It is sometimes seen in Gardner syndrome, after trauma, or after pregnancy.
- *Soft-tissue sarcoma:* Leiomyosarcoma, liposarcoma, fibrosarcoma, hemangiopericytoma, or malignant fibrous histiocytoma may present as a solitary mass without significant adenopathy.

## ■ Essential Facts

- GIST is the most common neoplasm of mesenchymal origin and may occur as a primary neoplasm of the mesentery or as metastasis to the mesentery.
- GIST is more common in the stomach, small bowel, and rectum.
- Metastases to the mesentery or omentum typically originate from a gastrointestinal (GI) tract primary GIST, most commonly in the stomach (65%), small intestine (25%), colon, or rectum. Fewer than 5% of GISTs originate in the esophagus.
- Immunoreactivity for KIT, a tyrosine kinase inhibitor, distinguishes GISTs from tumors originating from the mural smooth muscle of the GI tract, such as leiomyomas, leiomyosarcomas, neurofibromas, and schwannomas. A KIT inhibitor can treat this entity.

## ■ Other Imaging Findings

- CT typically shows a smoothly marginated mass with heterogeneous enhancement caused by cystic areas corresponding to necrosis, cystic degeneration, or hemorrhage.

## ✓ Pearls & ✗ Pitfalls

- ✓ Mesenteric fibromatosis is typically sporadic, occurs in young women, and may present with a solitary large mass or an infiltrative, local process causing bowel obstruction, perforation, and fistula. This entity does not metastasize.
- ✓ Inflammatory pseudotumor typically occurs in children and young adults as a result of local, chronic infection.
- ✓ Metastasis (particularly of GI origin) is always a consideration for a mesenteric mass, but it is less likely than the differential considerations listed in this case, given the solitary, well-circumscribed appearance.
- ✓ Lymphoma may present as large mesenteric mass, but the absence of other enlarged nodes makes lymphoma less likely.
- ✗ Because GISTs are treatable with surgery and a KIT inhibitor, failure to diagnose this entity can lead to unnecessary morbidity and mortality.

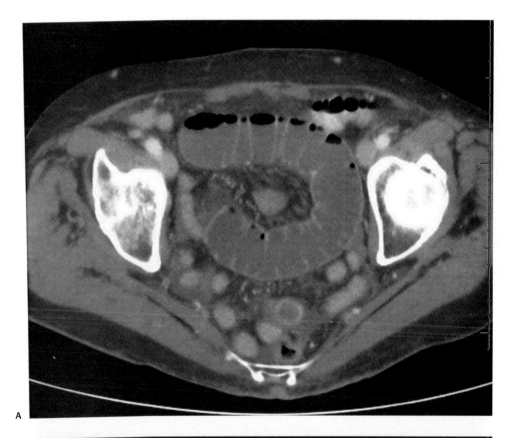

A

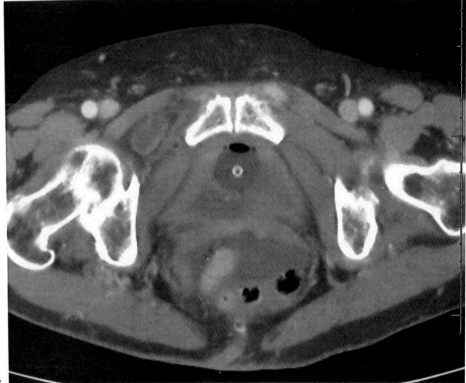

B

## ■ Clinical Presentation

A 91-year-old woman presents to the emergency department with intense abdominal pain.

### ■ Imaging Findings

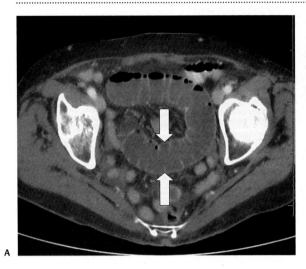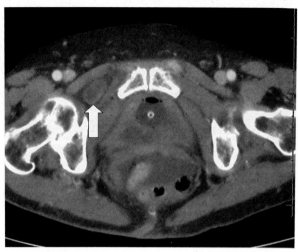

A                                                                                     B

**(A)** Contrast-enhanced computed tomography (CT) shows a markedly dilated loop of small bowel in the pelvis (*arrows*). **(B)** More caudal slice shows a segment of small bowel (*arrow*) between the external obturator and pectineus muscles.

### ■ Differential Diagnosis

- **Obturator foramen hernia:** This is the only diagnosis based on the finding of small-bowel obstruction, dilated small bowel, as well as a fluid-filled structure in the obturator foramen.

### ■ Essential Facts

- Pelvic external hernias are congenital, traumatic, or post-surgical herniations of pelvic contents through the pelvic wall or groin. They include inguinal, femoral, obturator, sciatic, and perineal hernias.
- Obturator hernia:
  - Usually right-sided in thin, elderly women
  - Herniation of bowel or genitourinary structures through the obturator canal between the pectineus and external obturator muscles
  - Obturator nerve compression may cause pain along the inner thigh (Howship-Romberg sign).
- Inguinal hernia:
  - CT clearly distinguishes direct (medial to inferior epigastric vessels) from indirect (lateral).
  - Indirect: Most common type; commonly causes bowel obstruction. It usually occurs in men and may contain peritoneal sac, bowel, and mesentery. Contents protrude down through the inguinal canal, anterior to the spermatic cord.
  - Direct: through the pelvic wall; rarely causes obstruction
- Femoral hernia:
  - Bowel and mesentery may herniate through the femoral canal. Commonly incarcerate and strangulate.
- Sciatic hernia:
  - Rare. Bowel or genitourinary structures herniate through the sciatic foramen to a potential space deep to the gluteus muscles.

- Perineal hernia:
  - Rare. Bowel or genitourinary structures herniate through the pelvic floor musculature and can be seen adjacent to the distal rectum.

### ■ Other Imaging Findings

- Radiograph may show herniated, fixed, gas-filled loops. In cases with marked dilatation terminating at the point of herniation, worry about incarceration or strangulation.
- CT is typically the best imaging modality to demonstrate the contents and extent of the hernia, the type of hernia, and the presence of complications, such as volvulus, obstruction, and ischemia.
- Ultrasound may be used to distinguish bowel from other structures containing fluid or air-fluid levels, such as abdominal wall or scrotal abscesses. Look for pathognomonic peristalsis.

### ✓ Pearls & ✗ Pitfalls

- ✓ Inguinal hernias occur above the pubic tubercle, and femoral hernias occur below the pubic tubercle.
- ✓ Abdominal external hernias include incisional, umbilical, ventral, spigelian, and lumbar hernias.
- ✗ In cases of incarcerated or volvulated hernia contents, do not miss pneumatosis indicating ischemic bowel!
- ✗ External hernias may appear as multiple fluid-filled structures or air-fluid levels, mimicking abdominal abscesses.

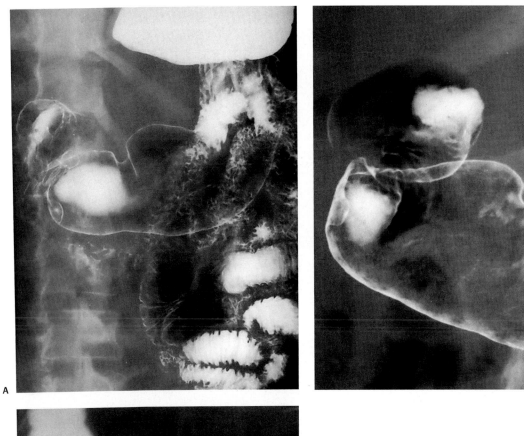

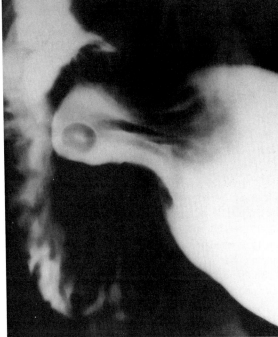

## Clinical Presentation

A 40-year-old man presents for an upper gastrointestinal barium study to evaluate chronic, mild midepigastric pain.

### ■ Imaging Findings

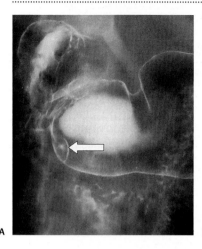
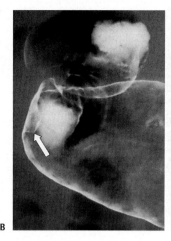
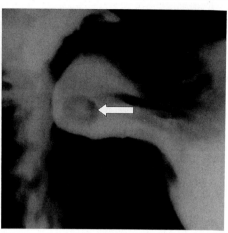

**(A)** Double-contrast barium study shows a submucosal lesion (*arrow*) in the gastric antrum, slightly in profile and slightly en face. A small collection of barium is seen within the center of the lesion. **(B)** Tangential view of the lesion (*arrow*) shows it to be focal and submucosal. **(C)** Single-contrast view en face shows the ovoid lesion with a central contrast collection (*arrow*).

### ■ Differential Diagnosis

- **Ectopic pancreatic rest:** This is the most likely diagnosis. It is a classic non-neoplastic cause of a single bull's-eye lesion.
- *Spindle cell or stromal tumor:* These tumors can be singular, submucosal, and centrally necrotic/ulcerated, including leiomyoma and gastrointestinal stromal tumor (GIST). These neoplasms are typically larger on presentation.
- *Primary malignancy:* These may be small, solitary, and ulcerated, such as adenocarcinoma, lymphoma, or carcinoid.
- *Eosinophilic granuloma:* This can present as a bull's-eye lesion.

### ■ Essential Facts

- Bull's-eye or target lesions of the GI tract on barium studies occur as a result of neoplastic masses or non-neoplastic tissue rests with central ulceration or umbilication.
- Bull's-eye lesions carry a broad differential diagnosis. Discriminating features include lesion size and multiplicity, as well as evidence of surrounding inflammation or neoplasm.
- Pancreatic rests of the stomach or small bowel may collect barium within a central, umbilicated duct.
- Peptic or aphthous ulcers are classically surrounded by a smoothly marginated mound of edematous mucosa (bull's-eye), but one would expect evidence of surrounding inflammation, such as rugal fold thickening.

### ■ Other Imaging Findings

- Computed tomography (CT) may narrow the differential to benign or malignant. Malignant signs include mural infiltration, distant metastases, and lymphadenopathy.

- Exophytic components of bull's-eye lesions not demonstrated on the barium study are clearly demonstrated on CT. Consider leiomyomas and GISTs.

### ✓ Pearls & ✗ Pitfalls

✓ Differential diagnosis of a bull's-eye lesion of the GI tract should begin with identification of the finding as single (see list above) or multiple, then progress to size and location.

✓ For multiple bull's-eye lesions, consider benign processes that cause aphthous ulcers and classic malignancies that metastasize to the GI tract and ulcerate (see "Differential Diagnosis").

✓ Regarding location, look for ectopic pancreatic rests, peptic ulcers, and breast metastases most commonly in the stomach and duodenum, Kaposi sarcoma and melanoma most commonly in the small bowel, and ulcerated lesions of Behçet syndrome most commonly in the terminal ileum and colon.

✓ Regarding size, pancreatic rests, peptic or aphthous ulcers, and Kaposi metastases are typically small. Other malignancies are variable. Spindle cell or stromal tumors can be quite large.

✓ Any cause of multiple bull's-eye lesions may present as a single lesion, including metastatic lesions from Kaposi sarcoma, melanoma, or breast, renal, or lung primaries.

✓ Kaposi sarcoma usually presents with a history of acquired immunodeficiency syndrome (AIDS) and cutaneous lesions. GI involvement is typically multifocal with ulcerated bull's-eye lesions in the stomach and small bowel.

✗ Clinical history should not be ignored. Does the patient have symptoms of peptic ulcer disease or a history of AIDS, a primary malignancy, or inflammatory bowel disease with aphthous ulcers?

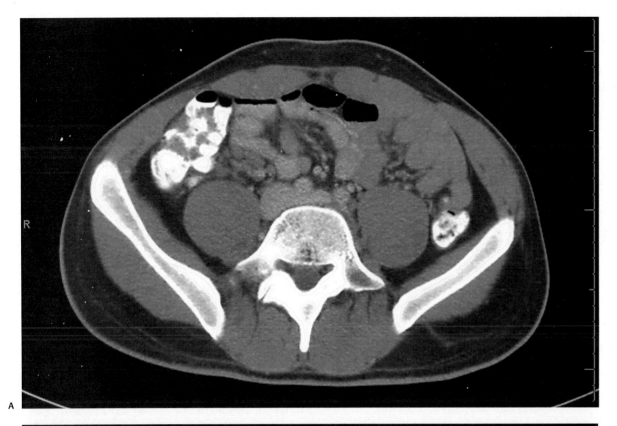

A

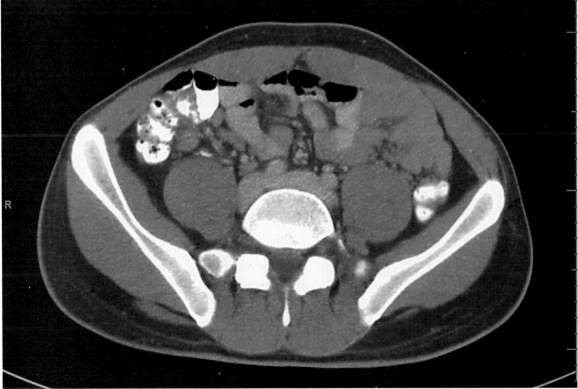

B

## ■ Clinical Presentation

A 23-year-old man presents with right lower quadrant pain and fever.

## ■ Imaging Findings

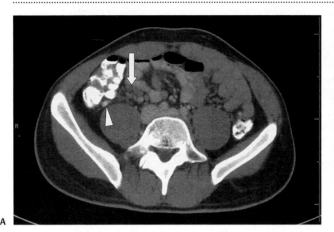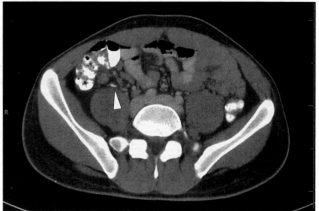

A                                                                                                                              B

**(A)** Contrast-enhanced computed tomography (CT) of the pelvis with oral contrast shows a cluster of enlarged mesenteric lymph nodes (*arrow*) in the right lower quadrant, adjacent to the cecum. The appendix fills with contrast (*arrowhead*). There is no cecal or appendiceal wall thickening or mesenteric fat stranding. **(B)** More caudal image shows contrast filling the appendix (*arrowhead*) without dilatation, mural thickening, or pericecal inflammatory changes.

## ■ Differential Diagnosis

- ***Mesenteric adenitis:*** This is the most likely diagnosis for a cluster of lymph nodes in the right lower quadrant without other evidence of inflammation or neoplasm.
- *Appendicitis:* This is an option that should be entertained, given the clinical history and findings. However, this diagnosis is unlikely, given the absence of appendiceal or periappendiceal abnormalities. Diverticulitis is less likely, given the absence of pericecal inflammation.
- *Neoplasm such as an occult colon carcinoma or lymphoma:* This may cause localized adenopathy, although the clinical history makes this diagnosis less likely. Endoscopy may be advisable.

## ■ Essential Facts

- This case reviews the possible considerations for focal mesenteric lymphadenopathy as an isolated finding.
- Mesenteric adenitis is a self-limited inflammation of the mesenteric lymph nodes, usually occurring in the right lower quadrant, as in this case.
- Clinical presentation may mimic that of appendicitis when it presents with focal abdominal pain, fever, and leukocytosis.
- Cross-sectional imaging may identify mesenteric adenitis by clustered, enlarged nodes combined with identification of a normal appendix. However, the normal appendix is misidentified or not identified in half of CT scans, making a definitive exclusion of appendicitis difficult in many cases.

- Occasionally, adjacent bowel wall thickening may be present in cases of mesenteric adenitis, further confusing the picture by raising suspicion for neoplasm, infection, or inflammation of the bowel as the primary process.
- Treatment of mesenteric adenitis typically involves the medical amelioration of symptoms. For equivocal cases, prophylactic antibiotic coverage and interval reimaging may be indicated.

## ■ Other Imaging Findings

- Look carefully for evidence of mild appendicitis, including wall thickening, diameter > 6 mm, periappendiceal fat stranding, or fluid and oral contrast pointing to the base of the unfilled appendix (arrowhead sign).

## ✓ Pearls & ✗ Pitfalls

- ✓ Crohn disease may cause focal adenopathy and bowel wall thickening in the absence of appendicitis, and subtle cases of new-onset Crohn disease may mimic mesenteric adenitis.
- ✗ Despite all efforts to definitively diagnose mesenteric adenitis, nonspecific imaging findings coupled with a suspicious clinical presentation often result in surgical resection of a normal appendix.

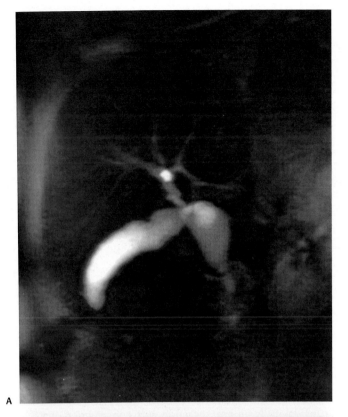

A

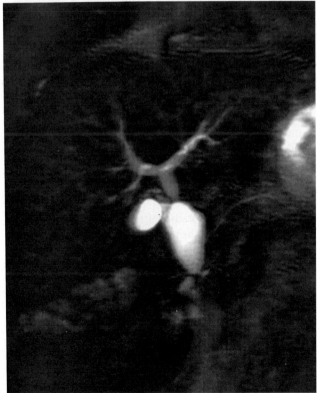

B

## ■ Clinical Presentation

A 29-year-old woman presents with abdominal pain and jaundice.

## ■ Imaging Findings

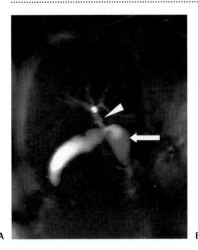 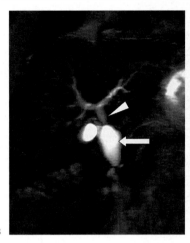 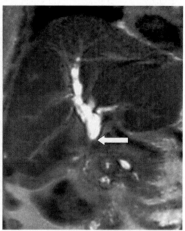

**(A)** Magnetic resonance cholangiopancreatography (MRCP) shows fusiform dilatation of the common bile duct (CBD; *arrow*) distal to the cystic duct. The common hepatic duct (*arrowhead*) is not dilated. **(B)** Oblique projection confirms fusiform dilatation of the CBD (*arrow*) with no dilatation of the remainder of the extrahepatic duct (*arrowhead*). **(C)** Magnetic resonance imaging after surgical resection and biliary-enteric anastomosis (*arrow*) shows persistent dilatation of the CBD despite normal serum bilirubin levels. This appearance may be a normal finding in any patient with a past history of chronic CBD obstruction.

## ■ Differential Diagnosis

- ***Choledochal cyst type IC:*** This is the most likely diagnosis, given the segmental extrahepatic duct dilatation.
- *CBD obstruction:* This may cause dilatation long after the obstruction is relieved; however, dilatation isolated to the CBD distal to the cystic duct is uncharacteristic.

## ■ Essential Facts

- Choledochal cysts are congenital defects believed to be caused by an anomalous junction of the CBD and pancreatic duct (PD) proximal to the normal location at the papilla. They are more common in women.
- As the sphincter of Oddi is separated from this anomalous junction, reflux of digestive pancreatic enzymes from the PD to the CBD occurs, resulting in gradual distension of the CBD.
- Clinical presentation: The classic triad of right upper quadrant (RUQ) colic, jaundice, and a palpable RUQ mass is present in only a minority of cases. Fever is often present. Most patients present in infancy or childhood.
- Todani types:
  - I:
    - A: saccular, majority of the extrahepatic CBD
    - B: saccular, limited segment of the CBD
    - C: fusiform, majority of the CBD
  - II: isolated diverticulum; often a narrow-necked CBD
  - III: duodenal wall, CBD (choledochocele)
  - IV:
    - A: multiple intrahepatic and extrahepatic
    - B: multiple extrahepatic

- V: multiple intrahepatic (Caroli pattern)
- Complications include rupture, bleeding, cholangitis, pancreatitis, stones, and malignancy.
- Treatment is surgical resection with construction of a biliary-enteric anastomosis, as in this case.

## ■ Other Imaging Findings

- Ultrasound is the best study, particularly for diagnosing choledochal cysts in a fetus, infant, or child.
- MRCP has become an excellent tool for identifying an anomalous junction of the CBD and PD without ionizing radiation.

## ✓ Pearls & ✗ Pitfalls

- ✓ Type I is the most common choledochal cyst.
- ✓ Malignancies associated with choledochal cysts include gallbladder adenocarcinoma and cholangiocarcinoma (in 10–20%).
- ✗ Always consider CBD or papillary obstruction when extrahepatic duct dilatation is encountered. Missing an obstructing lesion can have grave consequences!
- ✗ Non-neoplastic considerations include stones, ductal strictures, and pancreatitis.
- ✗ Neoplastic considerations include lymphoma and peri-ampullary neoplasms.

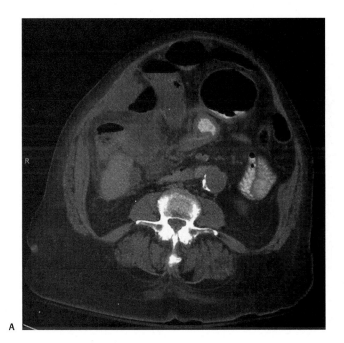

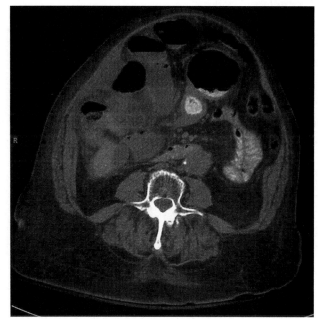

A

B

## Clinical Presentation

An 82-year-old presents with right upper quadrant pain.

### Further Work-up

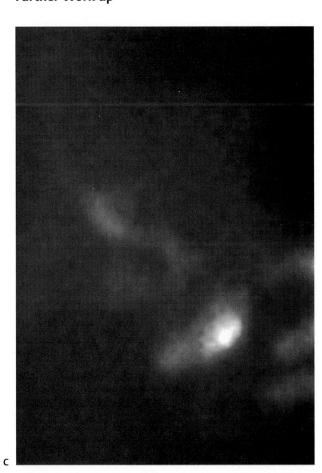

C

### ■ Imaging Findings

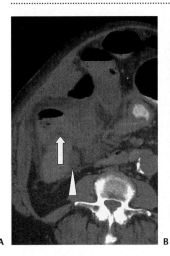 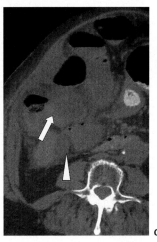 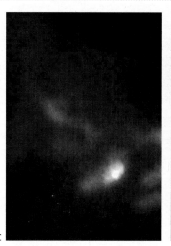 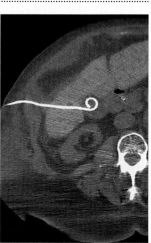

A    B    C    D

**(A,B)** Axial computed tomography images show infiltration of the fat surrounding the hepatic flexure (*arrows*), liver, and gallbladder. The fundus of the gallbladder, seen posteriorly (*arrowheads*), appears normal, but the body shows marked mural thickening. **(C)** Hepatobiliary iminodiacetic acid (HIDA) scan demonstrates nonfilling of the gallbladder, consistent with acute cholecystitis. **(D)** Successful treatment by cholecystostomy tube placement.

### ■ Differential Diagnosis

- **Cholecystitis:** This is the most likely choice, given the pericholecystic fat infiltration and gallbladder wall thickening.
- *Diverticulitis:* This is a possibility, given the infiltration of mesenteric fat adjacent to the hepatic flexure.
- *Appendicitis:* This can also mimic cholecystitis. The appendix can be as long as 20 cm and become inflamed in an unusual location, such as the right upper quadrant, left hemiabdomen, or pelvis.
- *Colitis:* Colitis affecting the right colon is possible but less likely as a diagnosis, given the relative absence of diffuse colonic wall thickening.

### ■ Essential Facts

- When faced with nonspecific findings affecting multiple organ systems:
  - Start with a broad differential diagnosis that includes affected systems and multiple disease categories.
  - Request additional clinical history to hone the differential diagnosis.
  - Suggest a follow-up study to further narrow the differential.
- When cholecystitis is in the differential for nonspecific imaging findings, recommend an HIDA scan as the definitive functional test.

### ✓ Pearls & ✗ Pitfalls

- ✓ Right-sided colitis is most commonly caused by ischemia or infection. Consider typhlitis, *Yersinia* infection, tuberculosis, amebiasis, *Salmonella* infection, and *Campylobacter* infection.
- ✗ For mesenteric fat stranding coupled with mural thickening of a hollow organ such as the bowel or gallbladder, do not forget to consider neoplastic possibilities:
  - Diverticulitis and colon carcinoma may be indistinguishable in 10% of cases. Signs of neoplasm include more marked wall thickening, polypoid mass, annular infiltration, and less pericolonic infiltration compared with diverticulitis.
  - Gallbladder carcinoma may show focal wall thickening, a polypoid mass, obliteration of the gallbladder lumen by a locally invasive mass, and enlargement of local lymph nodes.

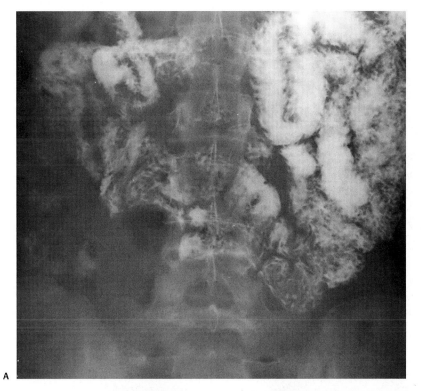

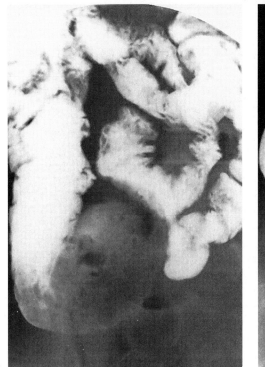

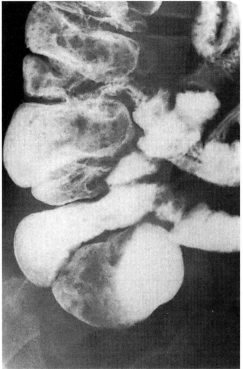

## ◼ Clinical Presentation

A 17-year-old girl presents with intermittent lower gastrointestinal bleeding.

## ■ Imaging Findings

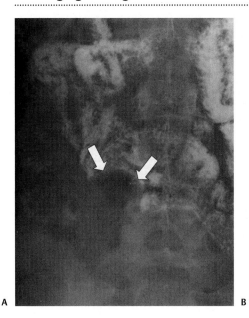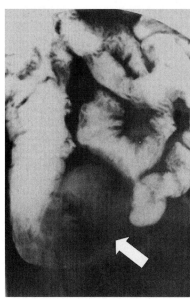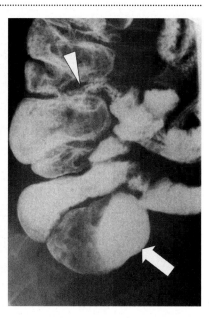

A                                                                          B                                                                          C

**(A)** Small-bowel follow-through shows an air-filled structure (*arrows*) in the right lower quadrant producing mass effect on the adjacent barium-filled small-bowel loops. **(B)** Compression view shows a wide-mouthed saccular structure (*arrow*) filled with debris and communicating with the terminal ileum. **(C)** Delayed view shows this saccular structure (*arrow*) along the terminal ileum some distance from the ileocecal valve (*arrowhead*). The sac is now filled with barium and debris.

## ■ Differential Diagnosis

- ***Meckel diverticulum (MD):*** This is the first consideration for a diverticulum of the terminal ileum in this location.
- *Small-bowel diverticulum (not Meckel):* Diverticula can occur anywhere in the small bowel, but most commonly in the duodenum.

## ■ Essential Facts

- MD occurs in 3% of the general population and is the most common congenital gastrointestinal anomaly. It is an antimesenteric ileal outpouching caused by failure of the omphalomesenteric duct to completely close.
- Clinical presentation varies by age. In children, bleeding results from ectopic mucosa causing peptic ulceration. Adults usually present with inflammation (diverticulitis) or obstruction. Pain may radiate to the right lower quadrant and mimic appendicitis.
- Complications include intussusception with an inverted MD as the lead point, bleeding, and diverticulitis, particularly when the diverticulum retains debris, as in this case. Rarely, MD can lead to small-bowel herniation or volvulus.

## ■ Other Imaging Findings

- Computed tomography (CT) commonly misses uncomplicated MD.
  - An enlarged diverticulum with retained debris, as in this case, should be visible, particularly when opacified with oral contrast.
  - An inverted diverticulum appears on CT as an intraluminal, fat-containing (mesentery) structure surrounded by bowel wall of soft-tissue density. The differential diagnosis includes lipoma.
- Technetium-99m pertechnetate scan should identify > 50% of MDs because of uptake by the ectopic gastric mucosa.
- CT enterography is gaining favor because it can identify complications such as intussusception. Specific features include arterial-phase enhancement caused by supply from the persistent omphalomesenteric artery.
- Angiography performed for bleeding may show extravasation or dense blush supplied by the omphalomesenteric artery.

## ✓ Pearls & ✗ Pitfalls

- ✓ MD often follows the "rule of 2s": 2% of people, 2 ft from the ileocecal valve, 2 in wide, and 2 years old. However, many of the patients are older than 2 years at presentation, as in this case.

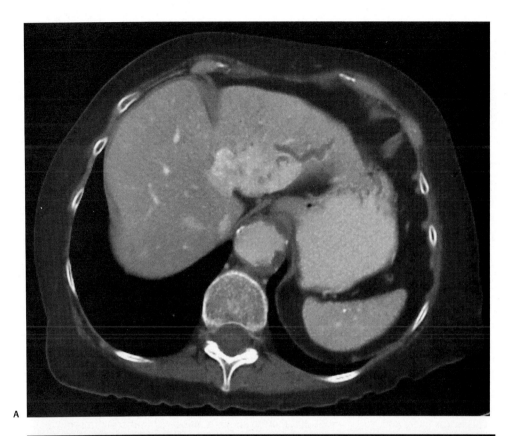

A

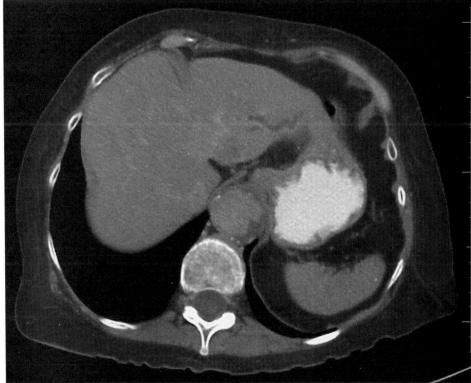

B

## Clinical Presentation

A 72-year-old woman with a known history of abdominal aortic aneurysm presents with nausea, vomiting, and jaundice.

### ▩ Imaging Findings

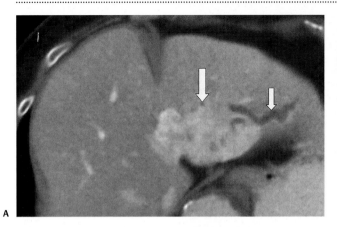 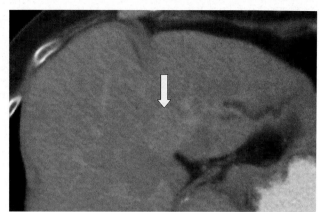

**A**          **B**

**(A)** Contrast-enhanced computed tomography (CT) shows avid arterial-phase enhancement of a single large mass in the left lobe of the liver, indistinctly marginated (*large arrow*) and causing intrahepatic bile duct dilatation (*small arrow*). Known aortic aneurysm is noted. **(B)** Delayed imaging (15 minutes) shows persistent mild enhancement (*arrow*) of the mass compared with the adjacent liver parenchyma.

### ▩ Differential Diagnosis

- **Intrahepatic cholangiocarcinoma (ICC):** This is strongly indicated by a single large, indistinctly marginated mass showing persistent enhancement on delayed imaging; intrahepatic duct dilatation supports this diagnosis.
- *Hepatocellular carcinoma (HCC):* This is less likely and would tend to lose contrast enhancement on delayed images.
- *Hypervascular metastasis:* Common sources include islet cell tumors, melanoma, and renal cell, breast, or lung carcinoma.

### ▩ Essential Facts

- ICC is adenocarcinoma originating from intrahepatic biliary epithelial cells. This tumor is the second most common hepatic primary malignancy after HCC.
- Predisposing factors for cholangiocarcinoma include chronic biliary infections or inflammation. Sources include pyogenic or parasitic infection, ulcerative colitis, choledochal cyst, cholangitis, and primary biliary cirrhosis.
- ICC is often solitary and large, lacks a capsule (indistinctly marginated), tends to infiltrate, and tends to cause fibrosis.
- Fibrosis leads to irregular margins, retraction of the liver capsule, and vascular invasion.

### ▩ Other Imaging Findings

- Ultrasound of ICCs may show bilateral or peripheral biliary dilatation, the absence of a discrete mass, a hyperechoic mass, and an abrupt transition from dilated to nondilated bile ducts.
- CT of ICC often shows a mass with indistinct margins, peripheral to central delayed enhancement, and persistent enhancement on delayed imaging. Look for retraction of the liver capsule.
- Cholangiography (endoscopic retrograde cholangiopancreatography, magnetic resonance cholangiopancreatography, or percutaneous transhepatic cholangiography) may show abrupt biliary obstruction or an irregularly marginated biliary stenosis with an abrupt, shelflike transition to a normal or dilated bile duct.

### ✓ Pearls & ✗ Pitfalls

- ✓ ICC tends to occur in patients with chronic or recurrent biliary infection or inflammation; HCC tends to occur in patients with cirrhosis and hepatitis.
- ✓ Smaller (< 3 cm) ICCs may enhance in a pattern similar to that of HCC. Larger lesions demonstrate the more characteristic enhancement with delayed washout.
- ✗ ICC may be difficult to distinguish from HCC on imaging studies, and biopsy is often necessary.
- ✗ The peripheral to central enhancement pattern of ICC is also seen with benign hemangiomas, but these entities are easy to distinguish.

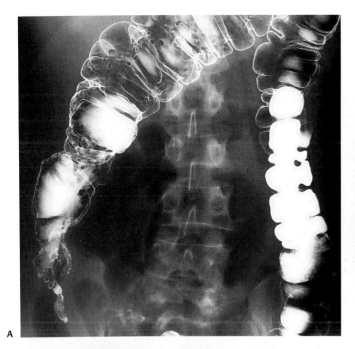

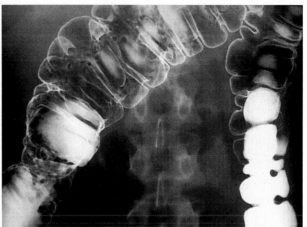

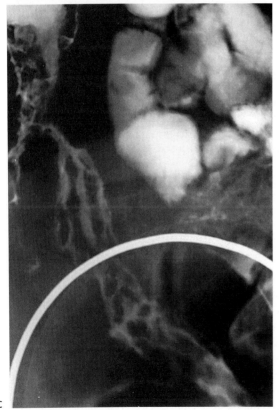

## Clinical Presentation

A 23-year-old man presents to the gastroenterology clinic with abdominal pain.

## ■ Imaging Findings

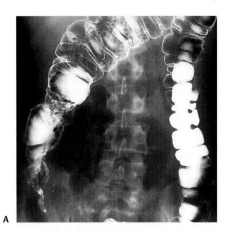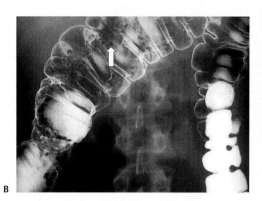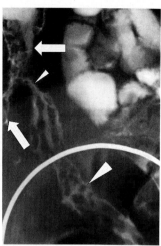

**(A)** Double-contrast barium enema shows a cone-shaped cecum and multiple polypoid lesions in the ascending and transverse colon. **(B)** Magnified view shows small, well-circumscribed polypoid lesions (*arrow*). **(C)** Compression view of the terminal ileum and cecum shows nodular, thickened ileal folds (*large arrowhead*); stricturing of the distal terminal ileum (*small arrowhead*); and a cone-shaped, nodular cecum (*arrows*).

### ■ Differential Diagnosis

- **Crohn disease (CD):** The constellation of multiple inflammatory filiform polyps; a cone-shaped, strictured cecum; and a strictured, nodular terminal ileum is most likely caused by CD.
- *Lymphoma:* This may be indistinguishable from CD in the terminal ileum and cecum but is less likely to cause luminal narrowing.
- *Tuberculosis:* This mimics CD in the terminal ileum and cecum and should be considered in the absence of a clinical history. Polyps are not characteristic.
- *Yersinia infection:* This is similar to CD in the terminal ileum and cecum. There are aphthous ulcers in both, but *Yersinia* infection resolves in 2 to 4 months with antibiotics. Polyps are not characteristic.

### ■ Essential Facts

- CD, or regional enteritis, is an inflammatory bowel disease of unknown etiology (most likely autoimmune) that usually presents in the first three decades.
- CD presents with skip lesions (skipped segments of bowel) and transmural involvement resulting in fistulae and fissures.
- Location is the terminal ileum in > 70%, but CD affects any portion of the bowel, from mouth to anus. The rectum and sigmoid are often spared (unlike in ulcerative colitis), but anal fissures and perirectal or perianal abscesses may be present.
- Gastrointestinal manifestations of CD:
  - Early: nodular, granular thickening; aphthous ulcers ("bull's-eye" or "target" lesions)

- More advanced: skip lesions; cobblestoning (serpiginous ulcers separated by edematous bowel); blunted small-bowel folds; pseudodiverticula; pseudopolyps (alternating hyperplastic and denuded mucosa); and the inflammatory polyps seen in this case
- Chronic: strictured, rigid enteric segments; risk for adenocarcinoma of the colon markedly increased

### ■ Other Imaging Findings

- Computed tomography:
  - Fissures and fistulae (especially enterocolic, enterocutaneous, anal-perineal); abscesses
  - "Creeping fat": extensive mesenteric fat separating small-bowel loops (may be seen on barium studies)
  - Markedly thickened bowel wall (up to 2 cm)

### ✓ Pearls & ✗ Pitfalls

- ✓ For strictures of both the terminal ileum and cecum, consider inflammatory bowel diseases (CD, ulcerative colitis with backwash ileitis); infections that mimic CD (tuberculosis, *Yersinia* infection, actinomycosis, histoplasmosis); and neoplasm (lymphoma).
- ✗ Tuberculosis and *Yersinia* infection can mimic CD in the terminal ileum and cecum.
- ✗ Amebiasis can cause a cone-shaped cecum but usually spares the terminal ileum, except in unusual cases with backwash ileitis.
- ✗ Ulcerative colitis can produce filiform polyps in the chronic stage and involve the terminal ileum via backwash ileitis.

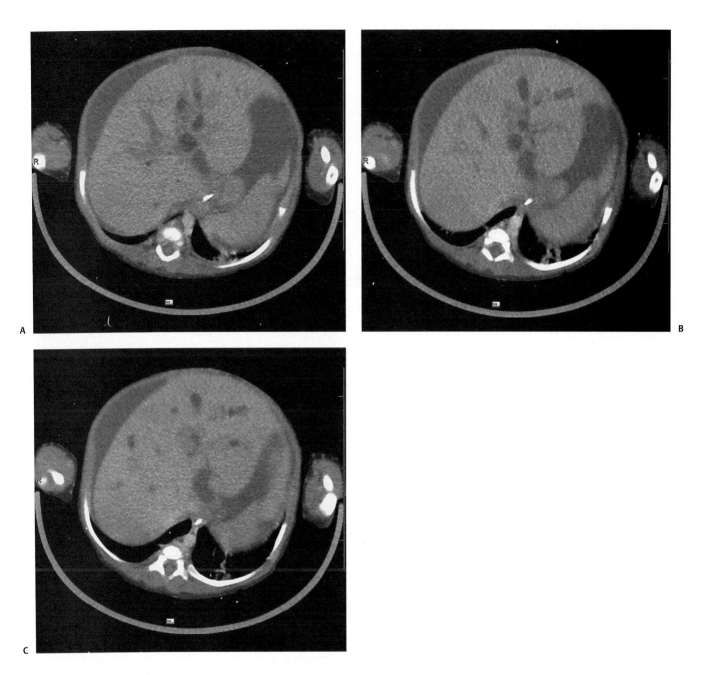

## Clinical Presentation

A 12-month-old boy presents with jaundice.

### ■ Imaging Findings

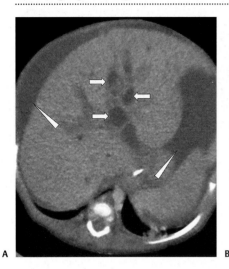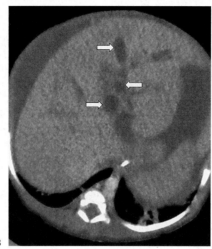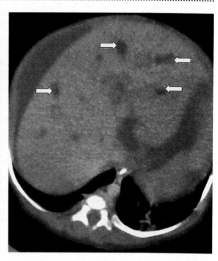

**(A–C)** Infused abdominal computed tomography (CT) shows multiple cystic structures (*arrows*) throughout the liver parenchyma, from the hilum to the periphery, in the general distribution of the bile ducts. Some of these structures may contain stone or sludge. The common bile duct is also dilated. Ascites is noted (*arrowheads*).

### ■ Differential Diagnosis

- *Caroli disease:* This is the most likely diagnosis for saccular and cystic structures within the liver parenchyma extending to the porta hepatis.
- *Biliary obstruction:* This typically causes uniform peripheral biliary dilatation rather than this focal, saccular appearance (from congenital causes such as biliary atresia).
- *Polycystic liver disease:* This is the principal differential possibility for the saccular appearance, particularly in severe cases with massively dilated peripheral ducts that are indistinguishable from large hepatic cysts. These are *not* present in this case.

### ■ Essential Facts

- Caroli disease is an autosomal-recessive disorder causing intrahepatic duct dilatation that is most commonly saccular, as in this case, but often variable in appearance.
- An associated condition is congenital hepatic fibrosis, which is believed to be caused by a similar embryologic defect: ductal plate malformation. Other associations include infantile polycystic kidney disease, medullary sponge kidney, and renal tubular ectasia.
- Cholangiocarcinoma occurs in patients with Caroli disease with a lifetime risk of < 10%. This risk is also associated with choledochal cysts.
- Cirrhosis is often absent, unlike in congenital cholestasis, which is commonly associated with cirrhosis. Uncommonly, cirrhosis may be a delayed complication of Caroli disease.

- Clinical presentation is jaundice, pain, fever, elevated bilirubin, and elevated liver transaminases indicating liver failure. Caroli disease may present at any age (typically from childhood to the 4th decade).
- CT may show saccular structures with intraluminal sludge, pus, or stones, reflecting a chronic obstructive process. Caroli disease may be limited to one or more segments or involve the entire liver. The common bile duct is dilated in the majority of cases.

### ■ Other Imaging Findings

- Ultrasound may show the classic finding of a central dot sign, which is characterized by dilated ducts with anechoic contents surrounding echogenic portal branches.

### ✓ Pearls & ✗ Pitfalls

- ✓ Complications of Caroli disease, such as abscess and stone formation, may be seen on imaging studies.
- ✓ Cholangiocarcinoma may be associated with Caroli disease and appears as focal enhancement or thickening of the duct wall, or as a mass within the parenchyma or duct lumen that enhances with delayed contrast washout.
- ✗ Duct dilatation is often more marked than in this case and often presents on imaging studies as large cysts of variable diameter that have no resemblance to intrahepatic ducts. Such cases may be indistinguishable from polycystic liver disease.

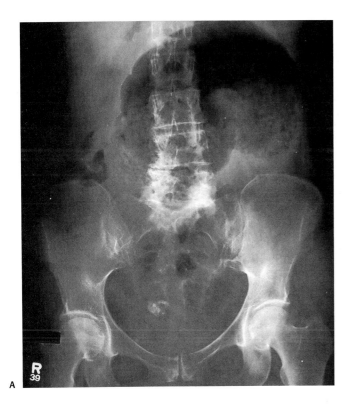

A

## Clinical Presentation

A 55-year-old woman presents with intense lower abdominal pain and distension.

## Further Work-up

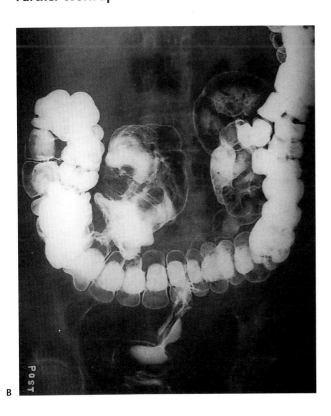

B

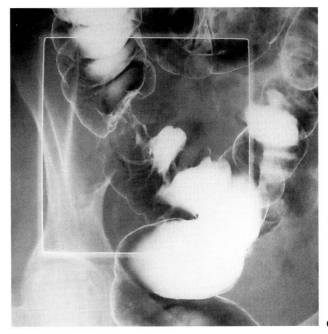

C

## ▇ Imaging Findings

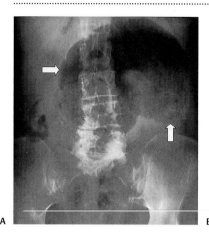 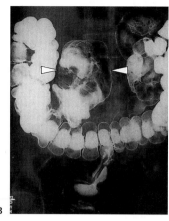 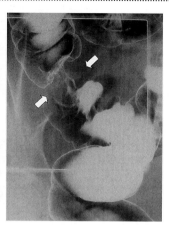

**(A)** Supine frontal abdominal radiograph shows markedly dilated middle to left bowel loop (*arrows*) with a caudal cleft, giving it the appearance of a coffee bean. No other dilated bowel is noted. **(B)** Single-contrast barium enema shows a dilated cecum projecting over the midline (*arrowheads*). After the radiograph was obtained, cecal dilatation diminished. **(C)** Compression view shows an apple-core lesion, consistent with colon carcinoma (*arrows*).

## ▇ Differential Diagnosis

- ***Cecal volvulus caused by colon carcinoma:*** This is the only possible diagnosis, given the cecal obstruction, the resolution before or during the barium enema, and the apple-core stricture.
- *Sigmoid volvulus:* This commonly presents with an inverted coffee-bean shape, as seen in this case. The barium study rules it out.

## ▇ Essential Facts

- The important feature of this case is the presence of two life-threatening diagnoses: cecal volvulus and colon cancer.
- Always look for a specific underlying cause of any bowel obstruction, particularly in cases of volvulus or intussusception.
- The radiographic findings of a dilated, air-filled midline structure and a decompressed distal colon are highly suggestive of colonic volvulus. A comma-shaped, enlarged cecum would be more specific.
- Cases of cecal volvulus may be iatrogenic (after surgery or colonoscopy); other causes include adhesion, atonic colon, pregnancy, and neoplasm, as in this case.
- Presentation is rapidly or insidiously increasing symptoms of abdominal pain, distension, and obstipation. Patients are younger than those with sigmoid volvulus (50s rather than 60s and older).

## ▇ Other Imaging Findings

- Radiographs:
  - Supine radiograph often shows a dilated midline loop in the midabdomen extending to the left upper quadrant.
  - Upright radiograph usually shows an air-fluid level.

- Single-contrast barium enema:
  - Barium enema may reduce volvulus (which possibly occurred in this case); instill contrast slowly to avoid perforation.
  - Round contrast collection (cecum) separated from the ascending colon by a transverse fold may be visible in cecal bascule.
  - Ischemic changes, such as mucosal thumbprinting, ulceration, and pneumatosis, may be visible.

## ✓ Pearls & ✗ Pitfalls

- ✓ A large, air-filled abdominal structure on plain film has a broad differential, including neoplasms, infections (pericolic abscess, amebiasis, tuberculosis, and schistosomiasis), strictures (ischemic, radiation, and inflammatory bowel), pseudo-obstruction, closed-loop small-bowel obstruction, and giant sigmoid diverticulum.
- ✓ A midline dilated loop with a coffee-bean shape on the abdominal radiograph would suggest sigmoid volvulus (barium enema rules it out).
- ✓ Ileosigmoid knot is a rare tangle of ileum, and sigmoid can have the radiographic appearance of colonic volvulus.
- ✓ Radiographs strongly suggest the diagnosis of colonic volvulus; computed tomography or single-contrast barium enema verifies the type.
- ✗ Barium enema is absolutely contraindicated in cases of pneumoperitoneum or mesenteric venous gas (gangrenous bowel requiring surgical resection)!

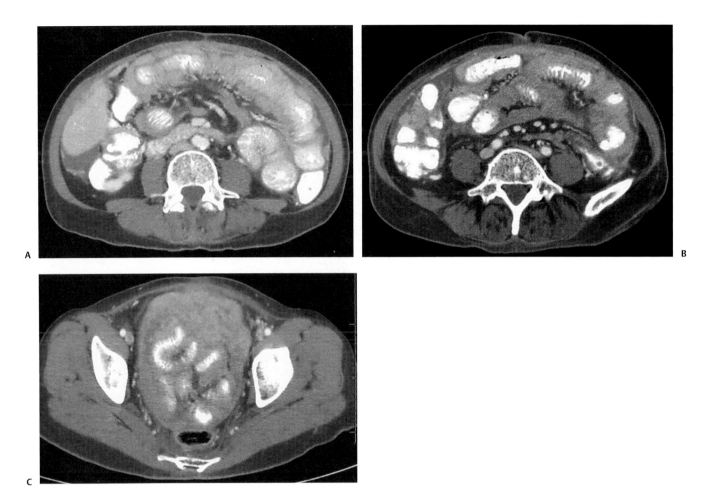

## ■ Clinical Presentation

A 56-year-old woman presents with nausea, vomiting, and increasing abdominal pain.

### ■ Imaging Findings

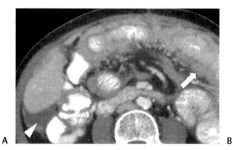 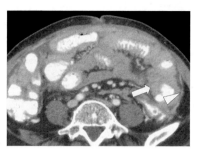 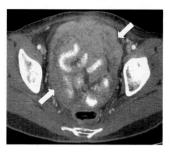

**(A)** Contrast-enhanced computed tomography (CT) shows extensive soft tissue infiltrating the mesenteric and omental fat (*arrow*) in the pelvis and abdomen with marked, diffuse bowel wall thickening. Minimal ascites is noted (*arrowhead*). **(B)** More caudal image again shows the infiltrating soft tissue (*arrow*) as well as peritoneal thickening and nodularity (*arrowhead*). **(C)** Pelvic image shows soft tissue (*arrows*) completely encasing the pelvic structures.

### ■ Differential Diagnosis

- ***Peritoneal malignant mesothelioma:*** This is the most likely diagnosis, as indicated by bowel wall thickening with soft-tissue infiltration of the mesenteric and omental fat (caking) and minimal ascites.
- *Primary peritoneal carcinoma (serous papillary carcinoma):* This option can cause omental caking, ascites, and enhancing, nodular thickening of the parietal peritoneum of the pelvis. However, normal-size ovaries suggest a peritoneal origin in these cases.
- *Peritoneal carcinomatosis:* This is typically more multifocal but can cause diffuse soft-tissue infiltration, nodularity, and peritoneal thickening as well as omental caking, depending on the primary.

### ■ Essential Facts

- Peritoneal mesothelioma is a rare primary tumor of the peritoneal mesothelium, typically occurring in patients in their 50s and 60s.
- Associated with asbestos exposure in 80% of cases, peritoneal mesothelioma is not typically associated with pleural mesothelioma.
- Histologic variants include desmoplastic, small cell, lymphohistiocytoid, and papillary.
- Imaging variants include diffuse malignant mesothelioma and cystic malignant mesothelioma.
- Prognosis is better than that of pleural mesothelioma, although median survival is still < 1 year.
- CT may show peritoneal thickening, nodules or masses, bowel encasement and bowel wall thickening, modest ascites, and masses or caking in the omentum and mesentery. Focal calcifications may be present.
- Ascites of malignant mesothelioma is typically minimal and has the attenuation of water, unlike the denser and more diffuse fluid associated with pseudomyxoma peritonei.

### ■ Other Imaging Findings

- Barium studies may show serosal implants as well as fixed and thickened bowel loops.

### ✓ Pearls & ✗ Pitfalls

- ✓ Infections such as tuberculosis and histoplasmosis rarely involve the peritoneum this diffusely and densely.
- ✓ Leiomyomatosis peritonealis disseminata may have the appearance of diffuse abdominal soft-tissue infiltration but is typically an incidental finding in young pregnant women with a history of contraceptive use and fibroids.
- ✓ Desmoplastic small round cell tumor can have this appearance due to desmoplastic reaction but typically occurs in younger patients and predominantly resides at or near the peritoneal surface.
- ✓ Pseudomyxoma peritonei can have a similar appearance to that of cystic malignant mesothelioma (diffuse, low-density material throughout the abdomen). Look for the characteristic semicircular calcifications of pseudomyxoma and an ovarian, pancreatic, or colonic primary.
- ✗ Disseminated infections can mimic diffuse peritoneal malignant mesothelioma.

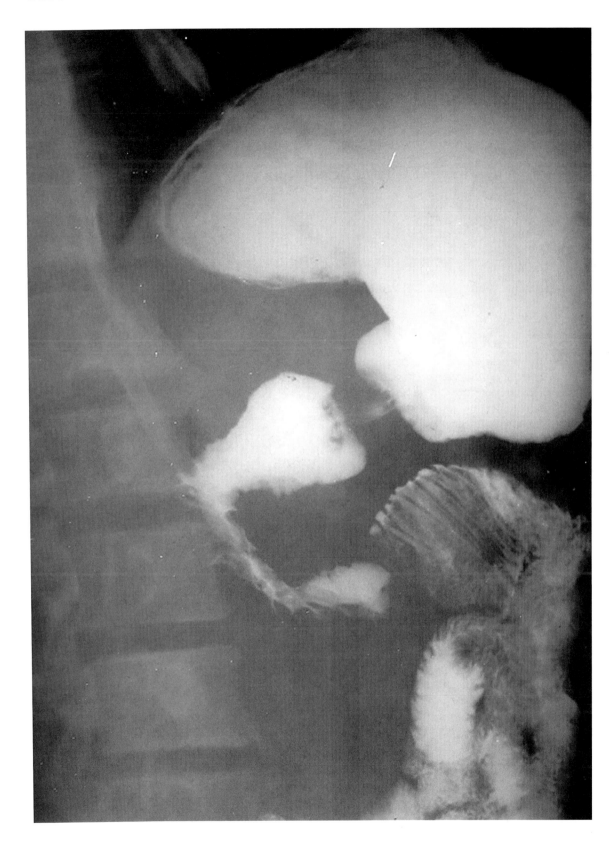

## Clinical Presentation

A 16-year-old boy is brought to the emergency department by his father. He complains of intense midepigastric abdominal pain.

### ■ Imaging Findings

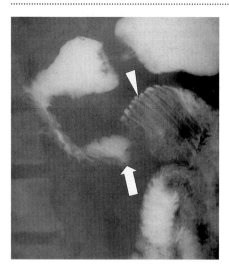

Single-contrast barium study shows an abrupt transition at the third portion from normal duodenum (*arrow*) to a segment with thin, stretched valvulae conniventes (*arrowhead*).

### ■ Differential Diagnosis

- ***Intramural duodenal hematoma:*** This is the most likely choice because of the coiled spring appearance of the duodenum on the barium study and the clinical history.
- *Intussusception:* This is a second option that can cause a coiled spring appearance, but it is unlikely to occur in fixed locations such as the duodenum.
- *Intraluminal mass:* This could have a similar appearance but would be unlikely, given the patient's age. Consider lipomas and windsock diverticula.

### ■ Essential Facts

- This case reviews the differential diagnosis for a coiled spring appearance of the small bowel.
- Intramural duodenal hematoma most commonly occurs with blunt trauma associated with motor vehicle accidents or child abuse.
- Predisposing factors include trauma, a bleeding diathesis, anticoagulants, and pancreatitis.
- Pathogenesis is crushing of the duodenum against the spine or at points of fixation, resulting in shearing of the mucosa from the submucosa and dissection of blood into the open submucosal space. This collection of blood can grow to efface or nearly efface the bowel lumen.
- Submucosal hematomas have been described elsewhere in the small bowel and in the large bowel.
- The coiled spring appearance of small bowel during a single-contrast barium study results when the intramural hematoma continues to expand and obliterates the lumen, stretching contrast-filled duodenal folds.
- Treatment is typically unnecessary because duodenal hematomas resolve over time. However, obstruction may occur, and the short-term placement of a nasogastric or Dobhoff tube and/or the administration of parenteral nutrition may be necessary. Surgery is rarely required.
- Intussusception is the classic alternative.

- The noncontrasted intussusceptum obliterates the contrasted intussuscipiens, producing the coiled spring appearance.
- This phenomenon is uncommon and more typically occurs beyond the ligament of Treitz as it relies on peristalsis of mobile bowel.
- Predisposing factors include celiac disease and lead points, both benign and neoplastic.

### ■ Other Imaging Findings

- Barium studies may show an eccentric, well-circumscribed intramural mass when the hematoma does not obliterate the entire duodenal lumen.
- Ultrasound may show a nonspecific cystic mass anteromedial to the kidney with variable echogenicity, depending on the degree of organization. Differential possibilities include duplication cysts, pseudocysts, renal cysts, necrotic or cystic neoplasm, and a duodenum filled with fluid.
- Computed tomography may show a homogeneously dense fluid collection that decreases in density over time and forms a dense outer capsule as it organizes.
- Magnetic resonance imaging may show the three-layered ring sign (concentric ring within; brighter than the hematoma on T1 and even brighter on T2).

### ✓ Pearls & ✗ Pitfalls

- ✓ The coiled spring appearance may result from any expansile, intraluminal filling defect that stretches the small-bowel folds.
- ✓ Differential diagnosis is ranked based on location (proximal or distal to the ligament of Treitz) and history (trauma causes hematoma, celiac disease causes intussusception).
- ✗ Do not miss associated signs of trauma, such as retroperitoneal hemorrhage, laceration of solid organs, and fractures!

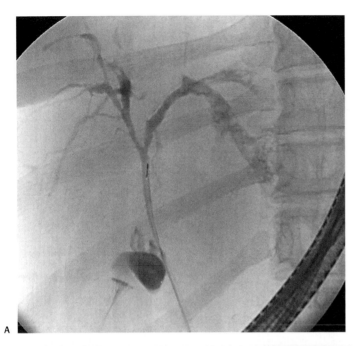

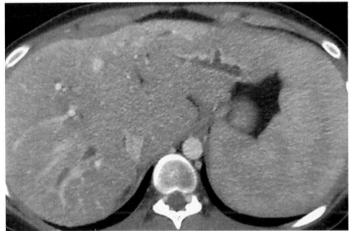

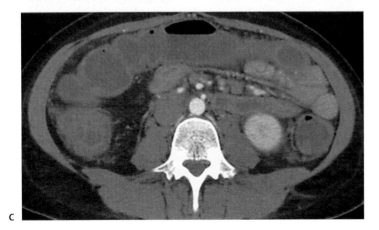

## Clinical Presentation

A 25-year-old woman presents with pruritus.

## ■ Imaging Findings

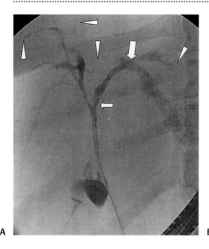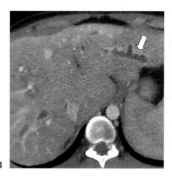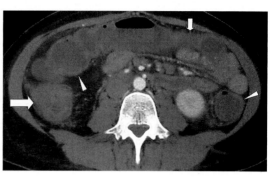

(A) Endoscopic cholangiography shows diffuse ductal irregularity involving the intrahepatic and extrahepatic ducts with pruning of the distal biliary tree (*arrowheads*), intraluminal filling defects (*large arrow*), and involvement of the ductal confluence (*small arrow*). (B) Contrast-enhanced computed tomography shows intrahepatic ductal dilatation with wall thickening and beading (*arrow*). (C) More caudal image shows marked wall thickening involving the cecum (*large arrow*), a diffusely featureless colon (*small arrow*), and diffuse moderate colonic wall thickening (*arrowheads*).

## ■ Differential Diagnosis

- ***Sclerosing cholangitis (SC):*** This diagnosis is strongly indicated by diffuse intra- and extrahepatic ductal irregularity, wall thickening, and dilatation, as well as beading and pruning.
- *Acute pyogenic cholangitis:* This is the less likely diagnosis as this is typically a post-obstructive condition caused by strictures, stones, and neoplasms. One would therefore expect more diffuse duct dilatation and an obstruction. In addition, the clinical presentation often involves acute bacteremia or frank sepsis.
- *Recurrent pyogenic cholangitis (oriental cholangiohepatitis):* This is a possibility, given the multiple findings characteristic of this condition (i.e., intraluminal filling defects that may represent the characteristic pigmented stones, ductal dilatation, and predominant involvement of the left lobe). It is common in Southeast Asians. It is caused by initial *Clonorchis sinensis* infection or ascariasis, followed by repeated bacterial infections.
- *Acquired immunodeficiency syndrome (AIDS)–related cholangiopathy:* This presents with diffuse ductal involvement and with all the features of SC. Cytomegalovirus or *Cryptosporidium* infection may or may not be present with AIDS and may cause findings similar to those of isolated infections without associated AIDS.

## ■ Essential Facts

- SC describes inflammation and sclerosis of the bile ducts. SC may be idiopathic (primary) or associated with other conditions and most commonly occurs in men younger than 45 years of age.
- Clinical presentation is progressive obstructive jaundice, fever, and pruritus.
- Associated conditions include ulcerative colitis (most commonly), Crohn disease (rarely), mediastinal and retroperitoneal fibrosis, and pancreatitis.
- Imaging findings include intra- and extrahepatic ductal involvement in the majority of cases; multifocal stenoses cause a beaded appearance, pruning of peripheral ducts, and ductal pseudo-diverticula (saccular outpouchings).
- Complications include cholangiocarcinoma in > 10% and biliary cirrhosis.

## ✓ Pearls & ✗ Pitfalls

- ✓ Primary biliary cirrhosis (PBC) is more common in women, unlike SC. The principal difference on imaging studies is that PBC is limited to intrahepatic ducts, whereas SC is isolated to intrahepatic ducts in only 20%. SC involves the common bile duct in nearly all cases.

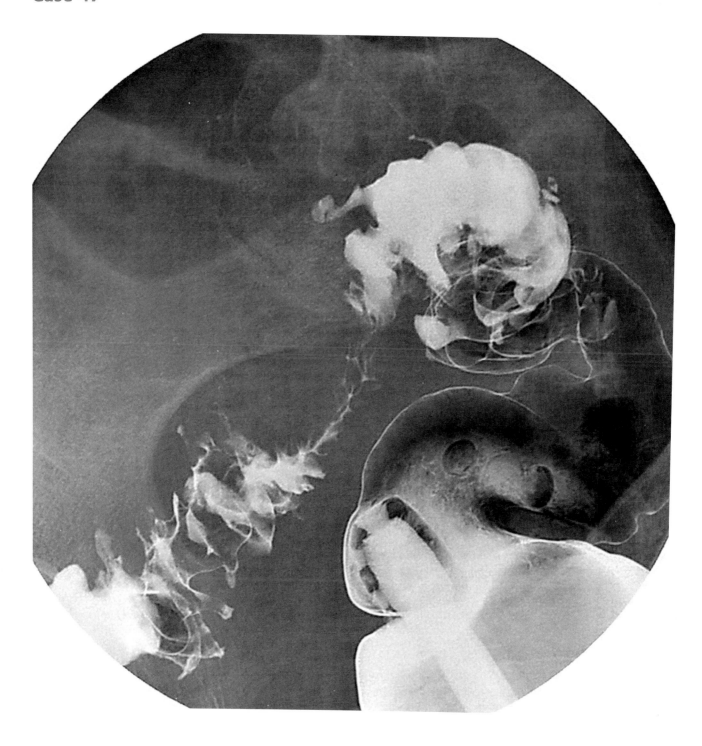

## ■ Clinical Presentation

An 83-year-old woman presents with fever after a long history of intermittent abdominal cramping and distension.

## ■ Imaging Findings

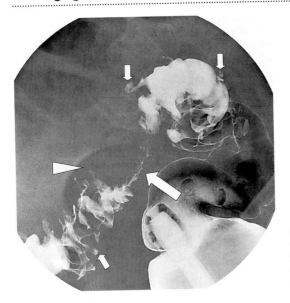

Barium enema shows a narrowed segment of sigmoid colon (*large arrow*) associated with mass effect along the superior margin and a subtle focus of barium extending toward a small extraluminal gas collection (*arrowhead*). Multiple sigmoid diverticula (*small arrows*) are present, and the transverse folds of the sigmoid colon are thickened, consistent with circular muscle hypertrophy.

## ■ Differential Diagnosis

- **Diverticulitis:** This is the most likely explanation for segmental sigmoid narrowing, sigmoid diverticula, and extrinsic mass effect associated with pericolonic gas (abscess). Diverticular disease without frank diverticulitis would be a consideration for thickened transverse folds in the absence of clinical signs of infection.
- *Colon adenocarcinoma:* This can cause focal "apple-core" strictures; however, the mucosa of the affected segment in this case appears intact. Necrotic tumors can cause pericolonic collections of gas and barium.
- *Crohn disease:* This is a third option that can cause a segmental colonic stricture, a pericolonic projection of barium (fissure or fistula), and a pericolonic gas collection (abscess).

## ■ Essential Facts

- When faced with an apple-core stricture of the colon on a barium enema, evaluate for mucosal abnormalities, diverticula, serosal abnormalities, mass effect, and the appearance of the surrounding colonic segments.
- Apple-core strictures can result from a variety of disease processes, including primary malignancies, serosal metastatic implants, infection of the colon or pericolonic space, endometriosis, and inflammatory bowel disease.
- Diverticular disease is indicated in this case by diverticulosis, a stricture with fold thickening consistent with chronic smooth-muscle hypertrophy, and relatively intact mucosa of the affected segment, reducing the likelihood of malignant stricture.

- Diverticulitis is indicated by features suggesting a pericolonic inflammatory process such as extrinsic mass effect and an extraluminal focus of barium and gas.
- Diverticulosis, diverticulitis, and diverticular disease most commonly affect the sigmoid colon.
- Any disease process causing colonic strictures can result in circumferential or asymmetric involvement. However, for circumferential narrowing, consider smooth-muscle hypertrophy from diverticular disease, ischemic stricture, infiltrating adenocarcinoma or lymphoma, and inflammatory bowel diseases.

## ✓ Pearls & ✗ Pitfalls

- ✓ Colon adenocarcinoma most commonly affects the rectosigmoid colon, making differentiation from diverticulitis difficult in some cases. On barium studies, malignancy usually causes mucosal abnormalities such as polyps, masses, and ulcerations.
- ✓ Crohn disease is similarly regional and transmural, and prone to abscess and fistula. Colonic involvement is more commonly right-sided.
- ✓ Serosal masses can cause extrinsic mass effect or scalloping with an intact mucosa. The sigmoid colon is commonly affected. Consider endometriosis and metastases from ovarian, colon, gastric, or pancreatic primaries.
- ✓ Abdominal masses such as lymphoma and mesenteric sarcomas can cause focal mass effect or narrowing of the colon.

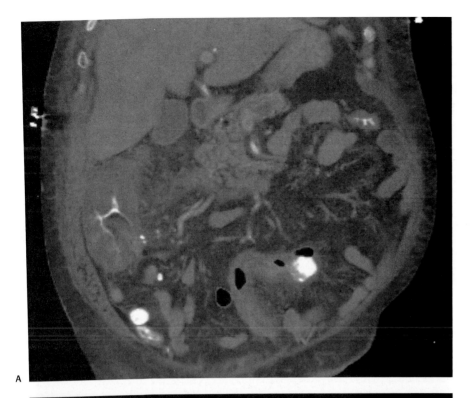

A

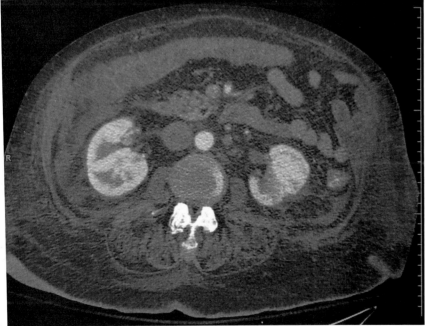

B

## Clinical Presentation

A 55-year-old man being treated for a kidney infection presents with diarrhea.

## ▦ Imaging Findings

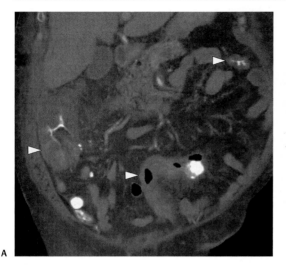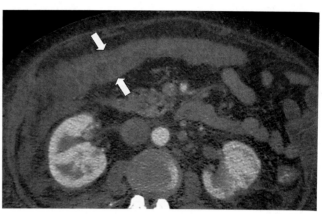

A                                                                                                                                                          B

**(A)** Contrast-enhanced computed tomography (CT) shows marked, diffuse circumferential thickening of the colon wall (*arrowheads*), trapped barium in mucosal folds, and mesenteric fat stranding. **(B)** Axial image shows circumferential thickening of the transverse colon (*arrows*) with obliteration of the lumen.

### ▦ Differential Diagnosis

- **Infection:** This is the most likely diagnosis, given that this patient has pseudomembranous colitis. Marked, diffuse, symmetric circumferential colon wall thickening with barium trapped in thick haustral folds is most typical of infections such as those caused by *Clostridium difficile* or cytomegalovirus (CMV; seen in acquired immunodeficiency syndrome). Also consider *Salmonella*, *Shigella*, or *Campylobacter* infection.
- **Inflammation:** This is a second choice as ulcerative colitis in the acute phase can have marked, diffuse colon wall thickening.
- **Ischemia:** This can be diffuse, symmetric, and circumferential—particularly in nonocclusive ischemia—but is often limited to a vascular distribution or to the watershed areas: the splenic flexure or sigmoid. Look for lack of enhancement.

### ▦ Essential Facts

- Pseudomembranous colitis is caused by the exuberant proliferation of *C. difficile* due to a reduction in the quantity of competing flora normally found in the colon. Pseudomembranes are exudates overlying edematous mucosa.
- Predisposing conditions include broad-spectrum antibiotics, hypoperfusion (shock, radiation, ischemia, dilatation from more distal obstruction), surgery, and debilitating diseases.
- Clinical presentation is abdominal pain, cramping, and diarrhea.
- Treatment is discontinuation of the offending antibiotic, treatment of causative conditions, and initiation of vancomycin and metronidazole.

### ▦ Other Imaging Findings

- Abdominal radiographs may show colonic wall thickening and thumbprinting; the small bowel may be distended.
- CT shows obliteration of the lumen due to marked circumferential wall thickening that distorts the normal haustral pattern (thickness of normal distended colon wall is < 3 mm). Colon wall enhances.
- Barium enema may show thumbprinting and barium invaginating into shaggy mucosa.

### ✓ Pearls & ✗ Pitfalls

- ✓ The type of colon wall thickening can help hone the differential diagnosis, although there is obviously much overlap in the appearance of diseases causing mural thickening.
- ✓ Eccentric, focal thickening suggests neoplasm. Look for lymph nodes and metastases. Alternative considerations include appendicitis and diverticulitis.
- ✓ Marked, diffuse circumferential thickening suggests infectious, inflammatory, or ischemic colitis. Consider pseudomembranous colitis, CMV, ulcerative colitis, or diffuse ischemia, as in the nonocclusive type (shock gut).
- ✓ Focal circumferential thickening suggests occlusive ischemia, Crohn disease, radiation, typhlitis, and occasionally neoplasms (think of lymphoma).
- ✗ Both pseudomembranous colitis and CMV colitis can be diffuse and cause pseudomembranes. For CMV, look for ulcers.
- ✗ Barium enema may be contraindicated in severe cases of pseudomembranous colitis (e.g., those associated with toxic megacolon).

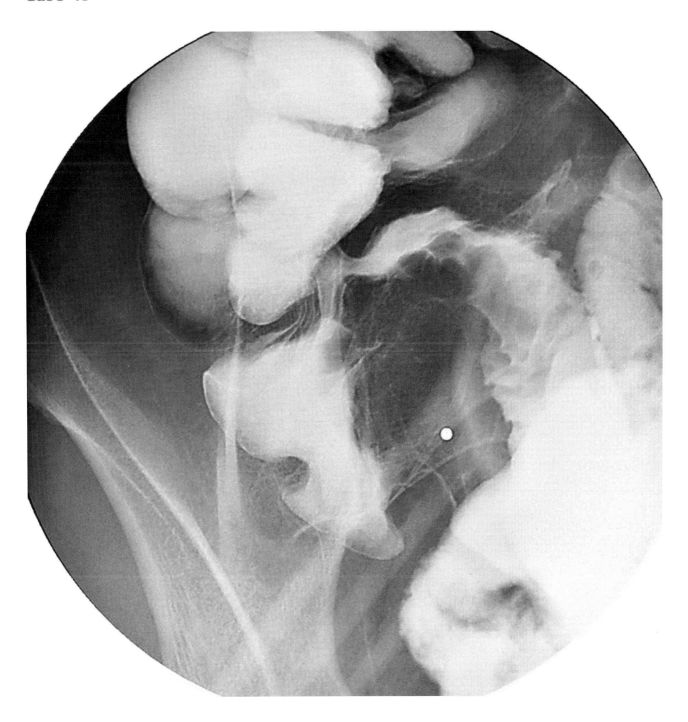

## Clinical Presentation

A 35-year-old man presents to the gastroenterology clinic with right lower quadrant abdominal pain.

■ **Imaging Findings**

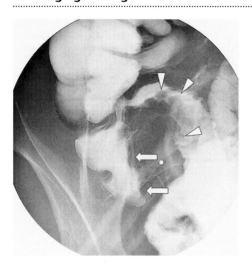

Compression view from a small-bowel series shows nodularity (*arrowheads*) along the inferior aspect of the terminal ileum (TI), with sparing of the superior aspect. The cecum demonstrates mucosal irregularity along the medial aspect (*arrows*), with sparing of the lateral aspect. The result is a C-shaped configuration of the TI and cecum and a cone shape of the cecum.

■ **Differential Diagnosis**

- **Lymphoma:** This is the top diagnosis, a classic cause of coned cecum with involvement of the TI.
- *Abscess from appendicitis or diverticulitis:* This diagnostic option can produce mass effect and inflammatory changes at the TI and cecum.
- *Crohn disease and tuberculosis:* These can also produce a coned cecum with TI involvement, but circumferential rather than eccentric involvement would be more common.

■ **Essential Facts**

- In this case, the white cell count and differential, history of fevers, and C-reactive protein level may distinguish between acute infection (abscess), chronic inflammation (Crohn disease), and lymphoma.
- Neoplasm or abscess is suggested by two factors: only one side of the TI and cecum is affected, and the TI and cecum appear displaced around a mass.
- Small-bowel lymphoma features:
  - It is the most common small-bowel malignancy (usually non-Hodgkin), and most small-bowel lymphomas occur in the TI.
  - It may be primary or secondary (celiac disease, Crohn disease, human immunodeficiency virus infection, other causes of immune compromise).
  - Long-segment infiltration is the most common pattern and often results in decreased or absent peristalsis and aneurysmal dilatation of the affected segment (disruption of the autonomic plexus). This finding may be associated with absence of small-bowel obstruction.
  - If the small-bowel neural plexus is intact, infiltration results in stricture and obstruction.

- Appendiceal lymphoma features:
  - Rare, but more commonly occurs as a first diagnosis than lymphoma of the small bowel
  - May mimic imaging signs and symptoms of appendicitis, including appendiceal wall thickening/dilatation and inflammation of the surrounding tissues and structures

■ **Other Imaging Findings**

- On imaging studies, small-bowel lymphoma can have a variety of appearances, including thickening or disruption of folds/wall, a focal polypoid mass, an ulcerating or cavitary mass, and segmental infiltration.
- Computed tomography typically shows larger mesenteric lymph nodes with small-bowel lymphoma compared with other small-bowel malignancies (normal abdominal lymph nodes are ≤ 11 mm). Lymph nodes may appear as a large confluent mass encasing other structures.

✓ **Pearls & ✗ Pitfalls**

- ✓ Adenocarcinoma of the cecum is a consideration for any case of mass effect and mucosal irregularity.
- ✓ Ulcerative colitis (UC) may cause TI disease with cecal involvement, but "backwash ileitis" is typically circumferential, not masslike, and associated with dilatation of the TI. Also, this entity occurs years after the diagnosis of UC, not as the presenting sign.
- ✓ Amebiasis can produce a coned cecum and occasionally an asymmetric mass (ameboma); the TI is typically not involved, and in this case, the characteristic aphthous ulcers are absent.
- ✓ *Yersinia* infection can cause a coned cecum.
- ✗ Do not miss perforation or ileocecal intussusception with small-bowel lymphoma!

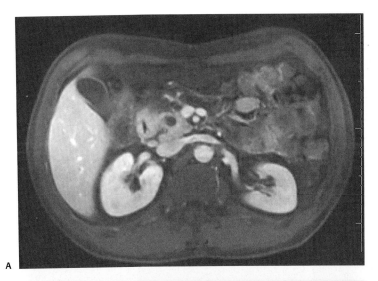

A

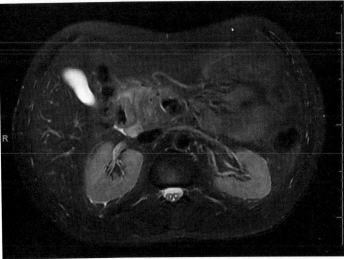

B

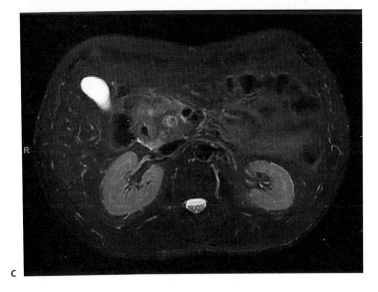

C

## ▨ Clinical Presentation

........................................................................................................................

A 40-year-old man presents with recurrent epigastric pain and a 20-lb weight loss.

## ■ Imaging Findings

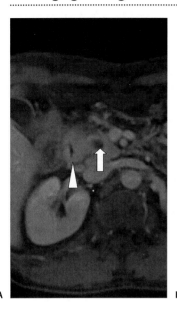 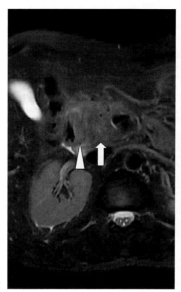 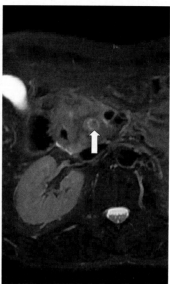

A      B      C

**(A)** T1-weighted magnetic resonance image (MRI) shows a focal lesion of low signal intensity (*arrow*) in the pancreatic head. There is focal thickening of the adjacent wall of the second portion of the duodenum (*arrowhead*). **(B)** T2-weighted image shows heterogeneous signal intensity in the pancreatic head (*arrow*) and focal duodenal wall thickening (*arrowhead*). There is increased signal in the peripancreatic tissues and in the pancreaticoduodenal groove, consistent with fluid and edema. **(C)** The focal lesion in the pancreatic head (*arrow*) is heterogeneously bright on T2.

## ■ Differential Diagnosis

- **Focal pancreatitis:** This diagnosis is the most likely explanation for peripancreatic fluid, duodenal wall thickening, and heterogeneous signal in the pancreatic head, as well as the focal lesion suspicious for a small pseudocyst or abscess.
- *Pancreatic neoplasm:* This is a diagnostic consideration for a focal lesion in the pancreatic head but is less likely, given the peripancreatic fluid, duodenal wall thickening, and abnormal signal in the pancreaticoduodenal groove—all more consistent with pancreatitis.
- *Duodenal adenocarcinoma:* This is an uncommon and unlikely choice in this case but can present as an infiltrating lesion in the enteric wall, with involvement of the pancreatic head.

## ■ Essential Facts

- Focal pancreatitis most commonly occurs in the pancreatic head or tail and may be difficult to distinguish from pancreatic carcinoma in some cases.
- In their early stages, both focal pancreatitis and pancreatic carcinoma can result in heterogeneously decreased signal intensity on T1 MRI due to fibrotic changes, both can weakly enhance because of mild hypervascularity, and both may show little change in size of the affected portion of the pancreas.
- Distinguishing early pancreatitis from carcinoma:
  - Pancreatitis more typically causes duodenal and gastric wall thickening due to inflammation.

- Pancreatitis tends to cause tapered narrowing of the distal common bile duct rather than an abrupt, shouldered transition.
- Pancreatitis presents with more acute clinical findings of fever, nausea, vomiting, and epigastric pain, although carcinoma can cause pancreatitis.
- Pancreatic carcinoma is associated with metastatic disease, local invasion, and more prominent lymphadenopathy.

## ✓ Pearls & ✗ Pitfalls

- ✓ Cystic lesions in the pancreas are most commonly pseudocysts (90%).
- ✓ Groove pancreatitis (this case) is an uncommon cause of focal pancreatitis that affects the groove between the pancreatic head, the duodenum, and the common bile duct. Mild changes in the pancreatic head and tapered narrowing of the common bile duct may be present, but the best sign is abnormal signal intensity (variable) in the pancreaticoduodenal groove.
- ✗ A focal cystic lesion in the pancreatic head may represent a pancreatic pseudocyst, a small abscess, or a cystic pancreatic neoplasm.
- ✗ Branch-type intraductal mucin-producing tumors may be indistinguishable from pseudocysts in some cases.
- ✗ The minimal enhancement or lack of enhancement common in pancreatic adenocarcinomas makes them difficult to distinguish from focal pancreatitis in some cases.

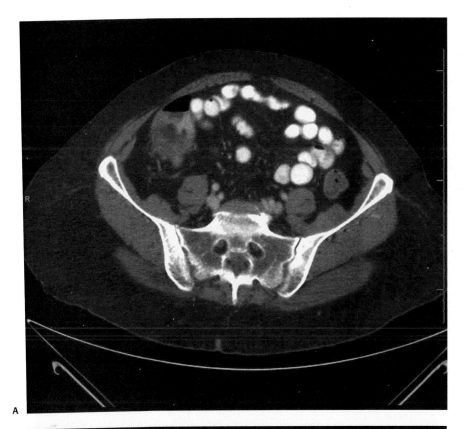

A

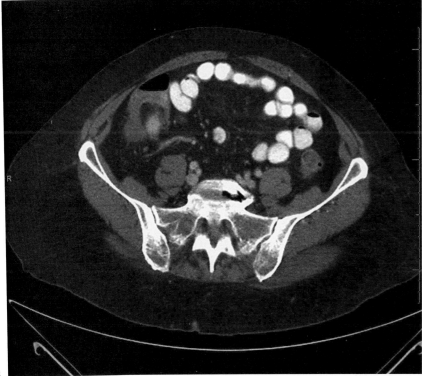

B

## Clinical Presentation

A 77-year-old woman presents with intermittent right lower quadrant pain.

### ■ Imaging Findings

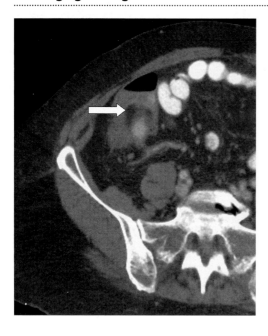

Contrast-enhanced computed tomography (CT) shows contrast within the terminal ileum abutting a fat-density mass (*arrow*) that projects into the lumen of the cecum.

### ■ Differential Diagnosis

- ***Ileocecal valve lipoma:*** This is the top diagnosis, indicated by a focal, fat-density mass that is not continuous with mesenteric fat.
- *Lipomatous infiltration:* This may have a similar appearance of fat density within the ileocecal valve.
- *Intussusception of the ileocecal type:* This can result in mesenteric fat projecting into the cecal lumen. This diagnosis is unlikely in this case because of the absence of continuity of mesenteric vessels and fat with this cecal fat-density structure, and the absence of the classic multilayer CT appearance of intussusception (see "Essential Facts").

### ■ Essential Facts

- This case reviews the differential diagnosis for a mass within the cecum containing fat. Maintain a good differential for ileocecal valve enlargement on barium studies or CT.
- The ileocecal valve is a polypoid structure (on barium studies) that is usually found on the medial cecum along the first haustral fold of the colon, but its location varies.
- Lipoma is the most common benign neoplasm of the ileocecal valve. This lesion is easily distinguished by its fat density on CT and by its variable shape, nodular appearance, and compressibility during barium studies.
- Lipomatous infiltration is non-neoplastic fat within the valve that is often more symmetric than lipoma, but often indistinguishable.
- CT of small-bowel intussusception without a lead point shows a sausage-shaped, kidney-shaped, or targetlike intraluminal mass. The classic finding of three layers of bowel wall and one layer of invaginated mesenteric fat and vessels may be present.

- Lipoma of the ileocecal valve can be a lead point for ileocecal intussusception. CT may show the multilayered appearance of intussusception and a fat-density mass at the end of the intussusceptum.

### ■ Other Imaging Findings

- Barium studies of the ileocecal valve show a variable size ranging from 1 to 4 cm, depending on the degree of cecal distension and the degree of partial prolapse of the ileum into the cecum (a normal finding not to be confused with intussusception).
- Barium studies rely on less specific indicators of an abnormal ileocecal valve, including the following: size > 4 cm during maximal cecal distension; incompetence of the valve during double-contrast studies; an irregular, lobulated contour; a carpet-like appearance (of villous adenoma); and abnormal contour of the adjacent cecal wall or haustral fold.

### ✓ Pearls & ✗ Pitfalls

- ✓ Benign lesions affecting the ileocecal valve include polypoid lesions, such as adenomas and lipomas, and nodular thickening from inflammatory bowel disease or infectious colitis. Consider *Yersinia* infection, tuberculosis, and amebiasis.
- ✓ Malignant lesions affecting the ileocecal valve include adenocarcinoma and lymphoma.

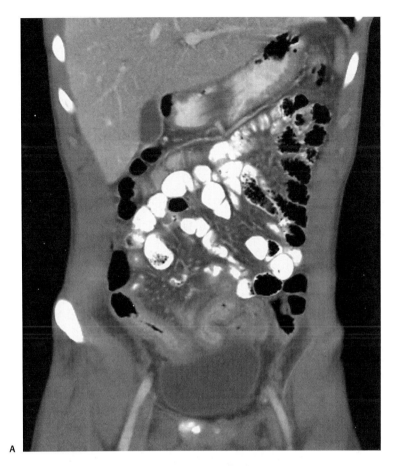

A

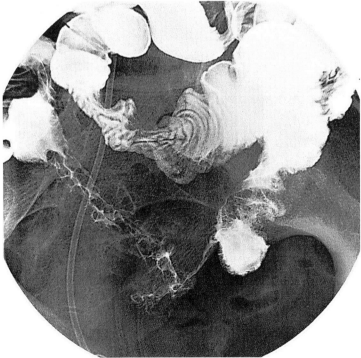

B

## Clinical Presentation

A 20-year-old man presents with a 1-year history of abdominal pain and diarrhea.

## ■ Imaging Findings

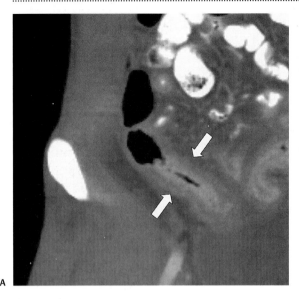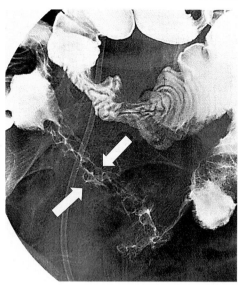

**(A)** Coronal reformatted infused computed tomography (CT) shows marked mural thickening of the distal small bowel (*arrows*) with a three-layer density pattern, consistent with the "fat halo" sign. In addition, there are dilatation and separation of the vasa recta of this segment along the mesenteric side, consistent with the "creeping fat" or "comb" sign. **(B)** Small-bowel follow-through shows a "cobblestone" appearance of barium (*arrows*) within the terminal ileum and an adjacent stricture ("string" sign).

## ■ Differential Diagnosis

- ***Crohn disease:*** This is the only diagnosis required for characteristic changes in the terminal ileum of cobblestoning, marked wall thickening, and mesenteric fat stranding with the creeping fat sign. Chronic stricture formation is also evident.
- *Infection:* Infections such as tuberculosis and *Yersinia* infection can involve the terminal ileum but are much less likely in this case.

## ■ Essential Facts

- Cobblestoning is an enteric feature seen in barium studies of patients with active Crohn disease and should not be confused with nodular fold thickening.
- Featureless, rigid strictures are associated with chronic changes of Crohn disease.
- Nodular fold thickening represents a less-advanced stage of active Crohn disease, when nodular folds are not yet effaced and the mucosa remains intact.
- Cobblestoning refers to larger, discrete filling defects surrounded by thin, intersecting, curvilinear collections of barium, as in this case.
  - The barium collections represent surrounding serpiginous, confluent, denuded mucosa.
  - The filling defects represent intact islands of remaining mucosa.

- Enhanced CT findings of Crohn disease may be variable, but evidence supporting this diagnosis in this patient includes the following:
  - Fat halo sign in the terminal ileum is a relatively specific indicator of Crohn disease, although chronic radiation enteritis can have this appearance. The finding is a three-layered wall consisting of a dense, thickened mucosal layer, a fat-density submucosal layer, and an outer, denser muscularis propria layer.
  - Creeping fat sign is a sign of inflammatory bowel disease caused by acute inflammation and hypervascularity. It is indicated by dilatation of the vasa recta and separation by perienteric fat deposition (also called comb sign).

## ✓ Pearls & ✗ Pitfalls

- ✓ Other types of small-bowel ulcerations include the following:
  - Aphthous ulcers, which are small, shallow ulcers with surrounding edema that occur with Crohn disease, tuberculosis, *Yersinia* infection, cytomegalovirus infection, herpes, and Behçet syndrome
  - Deep or linear ulcers, which occur with Crohn disease, ischemia, and radiation, as well as the infectious entities previously listed

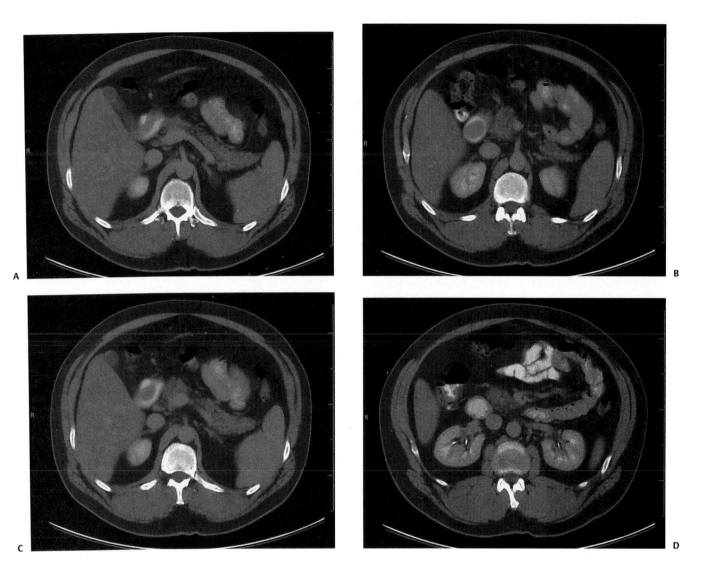

## Clinical Presentation

A 47-year-old man presents to the gastroenterology clinic with abdominal pain and recurrent gastrointestinal bleeding.

### ▓ Imaging Findings

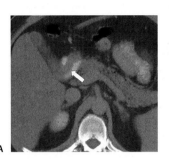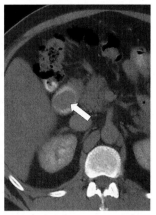

**(A)** Contrast-enhanced computed tomography (CT) shows a soft-tissue filling defect (*arrow*) originating from the immediate postbulbar duodenal wall. No adjacent wall thickening and no lymphadenopathy are present. **(B)** The soft-tissue filling defect (*arrow*) is polypoid and terminates in the distal descending duodenum.

### ▓ Differential Diagnosis

- *Adenoma:* This is the most likely diagnosis as it is commonly solitary and periampullary in origin.
- *Brunner gland hamartoma:* This is also solitary and well circumscribed, in the proximal duodenum, and either homogeneous or heterogeneous on CT, depending on the amount of cystic degeneration and fat.
- *Lymphoma:* This is a third option. It may be polypoid, but this presentation is less common than invasive lymphoma.
- *Adenocarcinoma:* This is most commonly periampullary or ampullary in origin and can be indistinguishable from benign adenoma in the early stages.

### ▓ Essential Facts

- Adenoma is an epithelial neoplasm consisting of dysplastic tubular, villous, or tubulovillous cells with the potential for malignant degeneration to adenocarcinoma.
- Associations include familial adenomatous polyposis (FAP) and hereditary nonpolyposis colon carcinoma (HNPCC)
- Imaging features: Adenoma is typically periampullary (80%) and solitary unless associated with FAP. The frequency of small-bowel adenomas increases proximally to distally, with > 20% duodenal, > 30% jejunal, and > 40% ileal.
- Adenocarcinoma of the small bowel is most common in the 6th decade, associated with the APC gene, and most common in the periampullary or ampullary region. Associations include chronic inflammatory diseases of the small bowel, FAP, HNPCC, neurofibromatosis type 1, and Peutz-Jeghers syndrome (< 3% develop adenocarcinoma of the gastrointestinal tract).
- Treatment is surgical resection as foci of malignant degeneration can be missed on endoscopic biopsy.

### ▓ Other Imaging Findings

- Features of malignant degeneration include adjacent duodenal wall thickening, biliary obstruction, infiltration of adjacent structures (fat, gallbladder, pancreas, common bile duct), and enlarged lymph nodes.

### ✓ Pearls & ✗ Pitfalls

- ✓ If a polyp is cystic, consider duplication cyst, choledochocele, hamartoma, or cystic degeneration of a neoplasm.
- ✓ If multiple polyps are present, consider Brunner gland hyperplasia, Peutz-Jeghers hamartomas, FAP adenomas, and lymphoid hyperplasia.
- ✓ If CT fails to localize the origin of the polyp to the duodenum, consider a gastric origin: prolapsed antral mucosa or prolapsed gastric neoplasm.
- ✓ Other considerations for small-bowel polyps include gastrointestinal stromal tumor, carcinoid, and metastasis.
- ✗ The origin of a duodenal polyp may be unknown, depending on the imaging quality and morphologic features such as size and effacement/infiltration of adjacent structures. Broaden the differential to include origin from adjacent structures as indicated.
- ✗ Evaluate for features of benignancy or malignancy before giving your differential diagnosis.

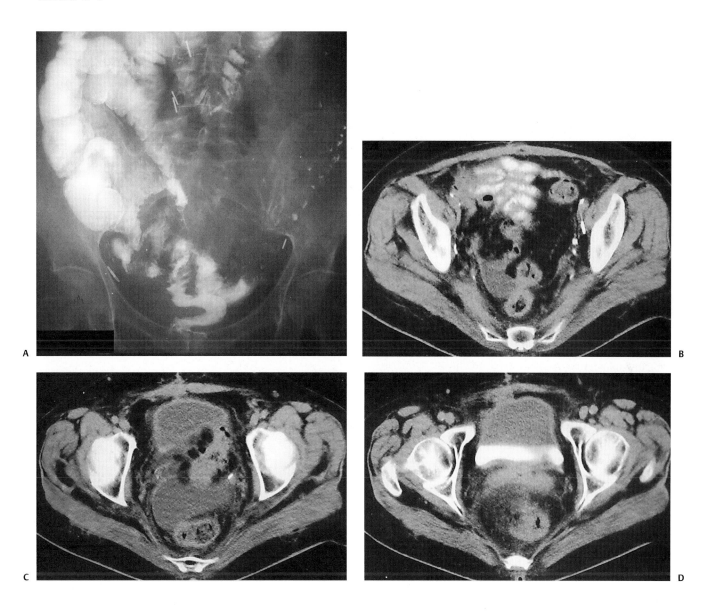

## Clinical Presentation

A 62-year-old woman presents with abdominal pain.

## ■ Imaging Findings

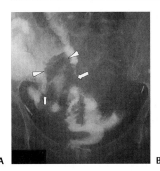 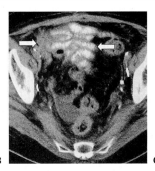 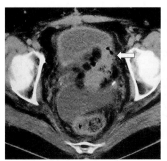 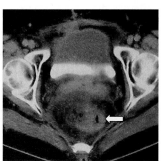

**(A)** Barium study shows fixed and separated small bowel (*arrowheads*), acute angulation of small bowel (*small arrow*), thickened folds, and stricture formation (*large arrow*). **(B)** Computed tomography (CT) shows multiple fixed, matted enteric loops (*arrows*) with adjacent soft-tissue infiltration, suggesting fibrosis. Bowel wall and fold thickening is also evident. **(C,D)** More caudal images show obliteration of the fat planes normally separating pelvic structures and rectosigmoid involvement (*arrows*).

## ■ Differential Diagnosis

- **Chronic radiation enteritis:** This is the top diagnosis, given the abdominal clips from prior surgery, tethering and angulation of small bowel, and involvement of nonadjacent structures, suggesting a distribution within a radiation portal (rectosigmoid colon, bladder, and small bowel).
- *Crohn disease:* This is worthy of consideration as it can cause mural thickening, mesenteric inflammation and fibrosis, and involvement of adjacent structures such as the urinary bladder with fistula formation (colovesicular or colovaginal), as well as stricturing, matting, tethering, and angulation of bowel.
- *Tuberculosis:* Tuberculosis can cause colitis and peritonitis with diffuse mesenteric fibrosis.

## ■ Essential Facts

- Radiation enteritis is endarteritis obliterans resulting in enteric ischemia due to radiation therapy. Changes may be acute or chronic.
- Ischemic bowel results from injury to arterioles that are too distal to allow perfusion by collateral arterial pathways.
- Acute radiation enteritis:
  - Presents during therapy as nausea, vomiting, and marked diarrhea caused by malabsorption resulting from sloughed mucosa.
  - Manifests on imaging studies as thickened bowel wall and folds.
- Chronic radiation enteritis:
  - May present months to years after therapy with diarrhea, bowel obstruction, and intestinal bleeding resulting from the combination of lost mucosa, fibrosis, and ulceration.

- Manifests on imaging studies as bowel wall thickening, separated loops of bowel, matted bowel loops, fixed strictures and angulations, and in severe cases featureless, ribbonlike bowel.

## ■ Other Imaging Findings

- Look for indiscriminate involvement of multiple structures within the radiation portal, such as the small bowel, colon, rectum, and urinary bladder. Generalized findings include fat stranding, obliteration of fat planes, adhesive fibrosis, and wall thickening.

## ✓ Pearls & ✗ Pitfalls

- ✓ Endometriosis can lead to tethering, kinking, and obstruction of small bowel in a female patient, but this entity was excluded in this patient as it typically presents during the childbearing years.
- ✓ Carcinoid with desmoplastic reaction can produce these radiographic findings, but involvement of small bowel and nonadjacent colon is unlikely.
- ✓ Lymphoma of the small bowel can cause fixed small-bowel loops due to bulky, confluent adenopathy and desmoplastic reaction.
- ✓ Retractile mesenteritis (sclerosing mesenteritis) can produce radiographic findings suggestive of focal fibrosis, but CT excludes this diagnosis by the absence of characteristic soft-tissue thickening centered at the mesenteric root and centralized, dense calcifications.
- ✓ Postoperative adhesions can cause fixed, angulated bowel loops due to fibrosis.

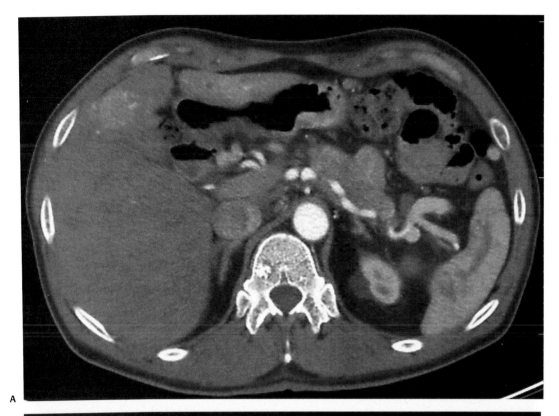

A

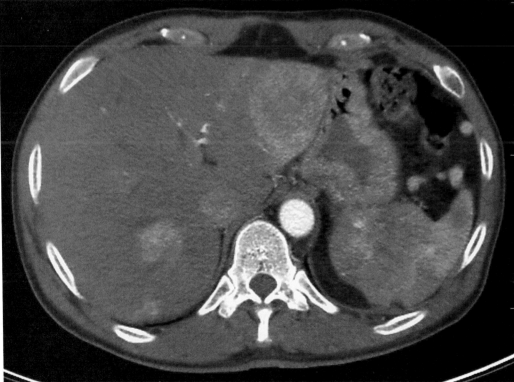

B

## Clinical Presentation

A 45-year-old woman presents with severe burning in the chest during meals. She is refractory to H2 antagonists and omeprazole.

## ■ Imaging Findings

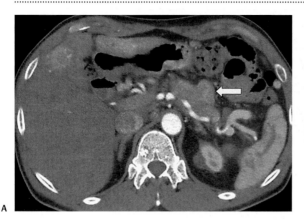 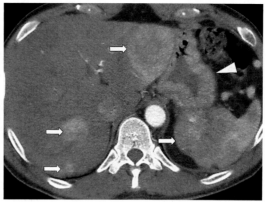

A                                                         B

**(A)** Arterial-phase contrast-enhanced computed tomography (CT) shows an enhancing exophytic mass involving the body and tail of the pancreas (*arrow*) and an enhancing mass within the medial segment of the left lobe of the liver. **(B)** Arterial-phase contrast-enhanced CT shows multiple enhancing masses within the spleen and liver (*arrows*) and marked thickening and enhancement of the gastric wall (*arrowhead*).

## ■ Differential Diagnosis

- **Gastrinoma:** This is the overwhelming choice as the diagnosis because of the classic findings of a small, homogeneously enhancing pancreatic tumor, hypervascular liver metastases, and gastric fold thickening due to hyperstimulation by a gastrin-secreting tumor.
- *Metastatic disease:* This is a distant second. Metastases from a hypervascular primary may have this appearance.
- *Pancreatic adenocarcinoma:* This is more typically hypovascular but is mentioned for the purposes of discussion.

## ■ Essential Facts

- Gastrinoma is a functional islet cell tumor that produces gastrin and is malignant in 60% of cases. Gastrinoma is extremely likely in this case, and other diagnoses are included only for the sake of discussion.
- Clinical presentation is classic: gastrin stimulates marked gastric hydrochloric acid release (Zollinger-Ellison syndrome) and causes hypersecretion and ulcers.
- Location is pancreas > duodenum > liver > lymph nodes.
- Gastrinoma is associated with multiple endocrine neoplasia type I syndrome, which is characterized by adenomas of the pituitary, parathyroid, and pancreas.
- Gastrinomas are typically small on presentation (< 2 cm), with dense, homogeneous enhancement on CT and no vascular encasement or necrosis. Malignant tumors often present with hepatic or nodal metastases.

## ■ Other Imaging Findings

- Upper gastrointestinal barium study: patients with Zollinger-Ellison syndrome have rugal fold thickening, multiple ulcers, and hypersecretion.
- Magnetic resonance imaging (MRI): gastrinomas have low to intermediate signal on T1 and usually very high signal on T2, and they are brightly enhancing.

## ✓ Pearls & ✗ Pitfalls

- ✓ In patients with functional islet cell tumors, the endocrinologist is typically able to diagnose the neoplasm by the clinical presentation.
- ✓ Imaging studies localize the tumor and any metastases to plan treatment.
- ✓ Gastrinoma may be localized by CT, MRI, or somatostatin receptor scintigraphy.
- ✓ Arterial-phase imaging in contrast-enhanced CT may be helpful because of intense early enhancement.
- ✓ Ectopic gastrinomas may occur in the stomach, duodenum, omentum, and ovaries.
- ✗ CT historically detects < 75% of gastrinomas because of their small size on presentation, but advances in scanner technology are likely to improve these numbers.
- ✗ Stimulation testing with selective arterial secretin injections and hepatic vein sampling may be necessary to make the diagnosis and localize the tumor in some cases.

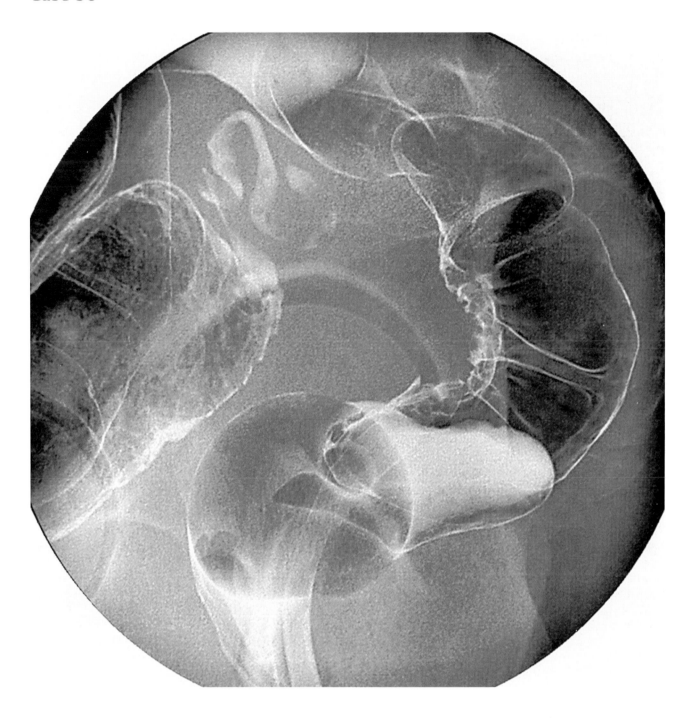

## Clinical Presentation

A 29-year-old woman presents with abdominal cramping.

## ■ Imaging Findings

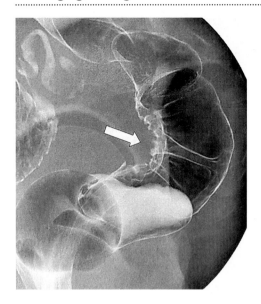

Lateral proctography shows plaquelike crenulations (*arrow*) of a focal portion of the anterior wall of the rectum, which appear to spare the mucosa but involve the serosa and submucosa. The remainder of the rectum appears normal.

## ■ Differential Diagnosis

- **Endometriosis:** This is the classic consideration for plaquelike crenulations of the anterior margin of the rectosigmoid colon in a young woman. This appearance is consistent with submucosal invasion by serosal implants of endometrium.
- *Abscesses:* This second diagnostic option can cause secondary inflammation of the anterior rectum. Infection can originate in the pelvis or secondarily spread to the cul-de-sac. Sources include diverticulitis, appendicitis, inflammatory bowel disease, and pelvic inflammatory disease causing tubo-ovarian abscess.
- *Serosal metastatic implants:* This is often a result of spread to the pouch of Douglas, usually from pancreatic, gastric, colonic, or appendiceal primaries.
- *Adjacent pelvic tumors:* Ovarian tumors or, less commonly, endometrial carcinoma should be considered.

## ■ Essential Facts

- Endometriosis is the proliferation of heterotopic endometrial tissue that spills into the abdominal cavity during menses.
- Rectosigmoid colon is the most commonly affected portion of bowel. Other common gastrointestinal locations include the small bowel, cecum, and appendix.
- Serosal implantation results in the local growth of endometrium. Two patterns typically result on barium studies:
  - Smoothly marginated foci of eccentric compression

- Invasion of the serosa and extension into the submucosa (usually with sparing of the mucosa), causing fibrosis and plaquelike crenulations or spiculations, as seen in this case
- Clinical presentation is typically pelvic pain and bowel obstruction, which cycles with the menses and stops during pregnancy. Rarely, involvement of the appendix causes acute appendicitis.

## ■ Other Imaging Findings

- Cross-sectional imaging and ultrasound may show multifocal, complex cystic masses that, when drained, contain dark brown liquid with debris ("chocolate" cysts).
- Small-bowel barium studies may show tethering, kinking, or angulation of bowel loops, occasionally with small-bowel obstruction.

## ✓ Pearls & ✗ Pitfalls

- ✓ Apple-core lesions mimicking primary colon carcinoma can result from rare transmural invasion to the mucosa by endometrium. Because both disease processes most commonly affect the rectosigmoid, imaging distinction may be difficult or impossible.
- ✗ Serosal metastases cause a similar appearance of mass effect and possible crenulations of the bowel wall by spreading through ascites to the small bowel, pelvis, and right paracolic gutter.

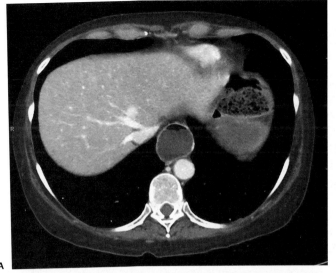

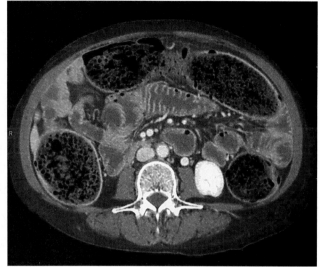

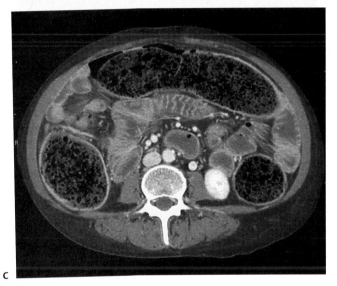

## Clinical Presentation

A 51-year-old woman presents with constipation.

### ■ Imaging Findings

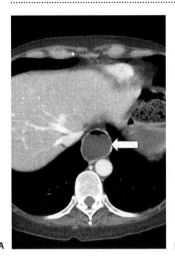
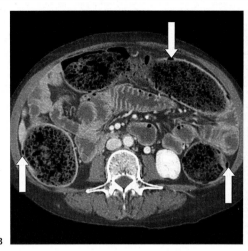
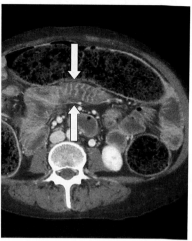

A                                         B                                         C

**(A)** Contrast-enhanced computed tomography (CT) shows marked dilatation of the esophagus (*arrow*). **(B)** Marked retention of fecal debris is noted throughout the colon, and gas is present within the colon wall (*arrows*) without associated mural thickening or mesenteric fat stranding, consistent with pneumatosis cystoides coli. **(C)** Stacks of thin, straight folds within the jejunum (*arrows*) are noted.

### ■ Differential Diagnosis

- ***Scleroderma:*** This is the diagnosis and is indicated by esophageal dilatation, marked fecal retention, the history of constipation, pneumatosis cystoides coli, and hidebound small-bowel folds.
- *Cystic fibrosis:* Cystic fibrosis can cause benign pneumatosis as well as retention of bowel contents. Marked esophageal dilatation is not characteristic.

### ■ Essential Facts

- The constellation of imaging findings and the clinical history of constipation in this case strongly indicate the diagnosis of scleroderma, or progressive systemic sclerosis.
- Scleroderma is thought to be an autoimmune collagen vascular disease that affects small vessels throughout the body, causing smooth-muscle atrophy, fibrosis, and collagen deposition. It involves the gastrointestinal tract in 90% and the esophagus in 80% of cases.
- Retention of food and debris in the esophagus is due to decreased peristalsis. This feature is increased in the supine position.
- Hidebound small bowel, as seen in this case, describes the increased frequency of thin, straight folds (typically jejunal), usually occurring after the onset of skin changes.
- Constipation occurs in up to half of patients with scleroderma, and CT may show marked retention of fecal debris, as in this case, and colonic dilatation with pseudosacculations.

### ■ Other Imaging Findings

- The CT findings associated with scleroderma in this case can also be detected on barium studies of the esophagus, small bowel, and colon.

### ✓ Pearls & ✗ Pitfalls

- ✓ Pneumatosis cystoides coli is a benign form of pneumatosis in which predominantly nitrogen gas collects in the subserosal space, often with a cystic or bleblike appearance. Predisposing conditions include steroid use, cystic fibrosis, scleroderma, and chronic obstructive pulmonary disease.
- ✗ Unnecessary surgery can be avoided by recognizing the benign nature of the findings, such as small-bowel dilatation and pneumatosis cystoides, associated with scleroderma. Correlation with the patient's clinical presentation is imperative.
- ✗ Barium impaction can be a serious, life-threatening consequence of barium use in radiologic studies of patients with scleroderma!

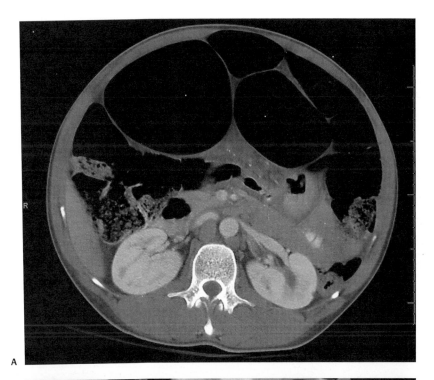

A

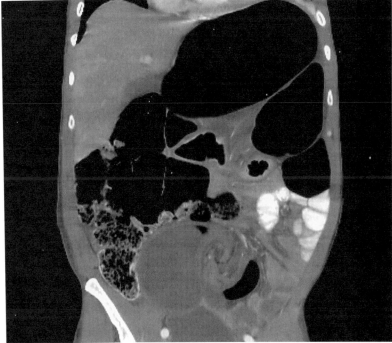

B

## Clinical Presentation

A 43-year-old man presents with intense lower abdominal pain and distension.

## ■ Imaging Findings

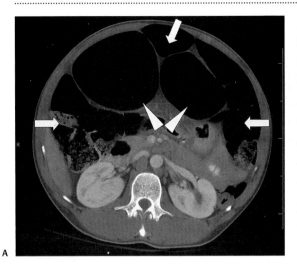 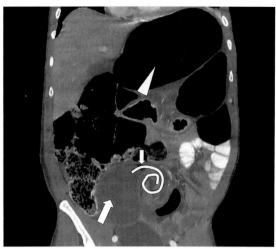

**(A)** Contrast-enhanced computed tomography (CT) shows two markedly dilated bowel segments (*arrowheads*) in the midabdomen surrounded by nondilated segments of ascending, transverse, and descending colon (*arrows*). **(B)** Coronal reformatted image shows a markedly dilated segment of bowel (*arrowhead*) with adjacent, nondilated transverse colon. A dilated, fluid-filled bowel segment (*large arrow*) in the lower abdomen terminates with a beaklike configuration (*small arrow*), followed by a whirl of mesenteric vessels and fat (*curved line*).

## ■ Differential Diagnosis

- **Sigmoid volvulus:** This diagnosis is strongly indicated by the CT findings of the whirl sign, the beak sign, and a markedly distended colonic segment with nondilated ascending, transverse, and descending colon.
- *Adhesion:* Beaklike tapering may result from adhesions due to surgery, radiation, infection, or inflammation. However, the whirl sign is uncharacteristic of this entity.

## ■ Essential Facts

- Sigmoid volvulus is abnormal rotation of the sigmoid colon, usually along the mesenteric (symptomatic) rather than the longitudinal (often asymptomatic) axis.
- Associations include redundant colon (common in patients on high-fiber diets) and constipation.
- Clinical presentation is vague low abdominal pain or acute, marked pain and distension with inability to pass flatus or stool; it is slightly more common in men, with two peaks: in children and in persons older than 50 years.
- CT with oral and rectal contrast is the least invasive study to rule out other diagnoses and evaluate the bowel wall for ischemic change:
  - *Beak sign* is abrupt rectosigmoid obstruction.
  - *Whirl sign* is twisted mesenteric vessels.
  - *Pseudotumor sign* is a fluid-filled, volvulated loop that looks like a soft-tissue mass.
- Do not miss the grave findings of portal venous gas or pneumatosis!

## ■ Other Imaging Findings

- Radiographs:
  - *Coffee bean sign* is classic: thickened, dilated colon in an inverted, ahaustral "U" shape.
  - *Double loop obstruction*: 50% of cases of sigmoid volvulus have a dilated distal colon, nondilated proximal colon with retained stool, and features of small-bowel obstruction.
  - Upright radiograph may show a dilated loop of colon: midline to left lower abdomen extending upward toward the right hemidiaphragm. The position of this dilated loop varies, however.
- Single-contrast barium enema:
  - This may diagnose *and* reduce the volvulus.
  - *Beak sign* may be present, often with a twist.
  - Do not miss mucosal thumbprinting and ulceration, indicating acute ischemia!

## ✓ Pearls & ✗ Pitfalls

- ✓ Closed-loop obstruction occurs when a segment of bowel is obstructed at both ends. This can develop in small or large bowel and most commonly results from volvulus, hernia, or an adhesion.
- ✓ In case of nonspecific colon obstruction, proceed to CT or single-contrast barium enema.
- ✗ Barium enema is contraindicated in patients with peritonitis, gangrenous bowel, or pneumoperitoneum.
- ✗ Supine radiograph may miss a fluid-filled loop. Upright view shows the air-fluid level.

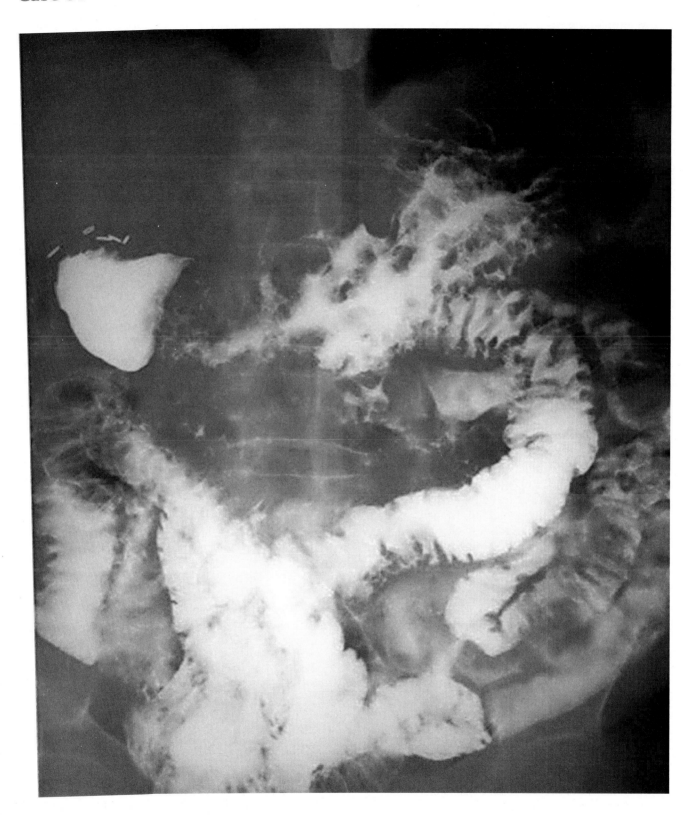

## Clinical Presentation

A 65-year-old woman presents with protein-losing enteropathy and marked weight loss.

## ■ Imaging Findings

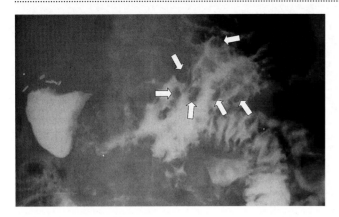

Single-contrast barium study demonstrates multiple polyps throughout the stomach (*arrows*) that are predominantly affecting the body. Rugal folds are thickened. Nodular thickening of the jejunal folds is also seen.

## ■ Differential Diagnosis

- ***Hyperplastic inflammatory (retention) polyps:*** This top diagnosis is associated with Canada-Cronkhite syndrome, which is rare. It has a distinctive clinical presentation consistent with this patient's history. This patient's age is also consistent with Canada-Cronkhite syndrome.
- *Hamartomatous polyps:* These are the second choice as they are typically multiple and tend to spare the antrum, as in this case. They occur as part of Peutz-Jeghers syndrome, familial polyposis, or Cowden syndrome.
- *Hyperplastic gastric polyps:* This is the third option because of the clinical presentation suggesting chronic gastritis, the high incidence of this type of gastric polyp (70–90% of gastric polyps), and the preponderance of polyps in the gastric body of this patient. Small-bowel involvement makes this diagnosis less likely.
- *Adenomatous polyps:* These are less likely as they are typically solitary and antral, and therefore listed below hamartomas.

## ■ Essential Facts

- The differential diagnosis for multiple gastric polyps is best remembered and presented by histologic polyp type, with names of the polyposis syndromes added as you progress through the list.
- Canada-Cronkhite:
  - Hyperplastic inflammatory retention polyps: stomach, small bowel, colon
  - Decades 5 to 8; marked weight loss, protein-losing enteropathy, diarrhea, peripheral edema, anemia
  - Loss of hair and nails, cutaneous hyperpigmentation
- Peutz-Jeghers:
  - Hamartomas: stomach, small bowel, colon
  - Decades 2 to 3; recurrent abdominal pain (intussusceptions of small bowel), orocutaneous hyperpigmentation

  - Increased risk for carcinoma of the colon, small bowel, breast, ovaries, pancreas
- Hyperplastic gastric polyposis:
  - Hyperplastic polyps constitute up to 90% of gastric polyps.
  - Any age; results from chronic gastritis
  - Polyps vary in size (usually < 1 cm), may be multiple, and may be located anywhere in the stomach, predominantly affecting the body.
- Familial polyposis:
  - Adenomas and hamartomas of the stomach have been described, but colon polyps are adenomas.
  - Risk for carcinomas of the thyroid (papillary), upper gastrointestinal tract, small bowel, and colon
  - Decades 3 to 4; desmoid tumors, osteomas (skull, mandible), dental anomalies
  - Turcot syndrome may be an extremely rare variant of familial polyposis with gliomas and/or medulloblastoma.
- Cowden:
  - Hamartomas of the tongue, skin, and entire gastrointestinal tract
  - Autosomal-dominant and extremely rare
  - Increased risk for thyroid and breast carcinoma (50% chance of breast cancer)

## ✓ Pearls & ✗ Pitfalls

- ✓ Organize any discussion of gastric polyps based on the history, number, location, and histologic types.
- ✓ Gastric polyps are usually hyperplastic and caused by chronic gastritis.
- ✓ The second consideration should be adenoma (if solitary, large, and antral) or hamartoma (if multiple).
- ✗ Note that both gastric adenomas and hamartomas have been described with familial polyposis.

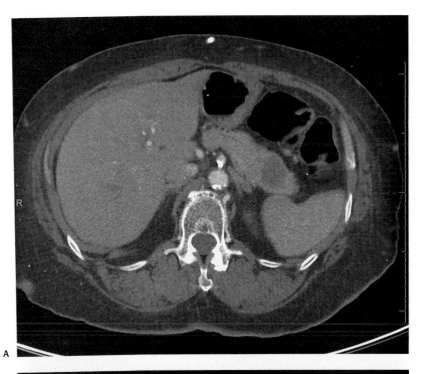

A

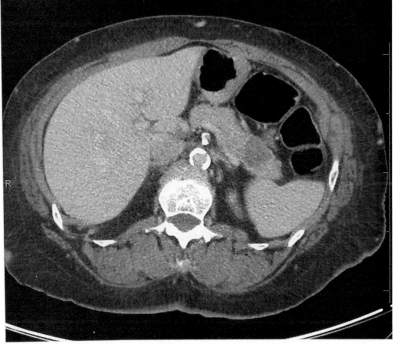

B

### ■ Clinical Presentation

A 61-year-old man presents with chronic back pain.

### ■ Imaging Findings

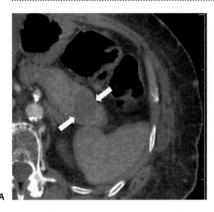 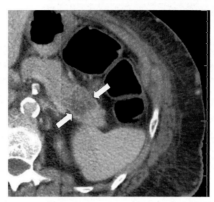

**(A)** Contrast-enhanced computed tomography (CT) in the arterial phase shows a well-circumscribed, hypodense mass (*arrows*) with punctate calcifications in the tail of the pancreas, without associated lymphadenopathy or infiltration of adjacent structures. **(B)** Venous-phase image shows a moderately enhancing mass (*arrows*) with a granular appearance suggesting multiple small cysts, internal septations, and the hint of a central scar.

### ■ Differential Diagnosis

- *Microcystic adenoma:* This is the most likely diagnosis, suggested by the subtle appearance of multiple small cysts, septa, and a central scar. A demonstration of stability on serial CT scans would further suggest this benign entity.
- *Pancreatic adenocarcinoma:* This is the worst-case scenario for any pancreatic mass, but no supportive findings, such as obliteration or stranding of peripancreatic fat, local extension into the splenic hilum, contiguous organ invasion, splenic venous obstruction or invasion, and distant metastasis, are visible.
- *Hemorrhagic pseudocyst, abscess, or necrosis:* Fluid collections or necrosis could have this appearance, although moderate central enhancement makes these entities less likely. Correlation with a clinical history of infection or pancreatitis is imperative.

### ■ Essential Facts

- Microcystic adenoma is a benign tumor made up of glycogen-rich cuboidal epithelium lining small cysts that contain protein-rich fluid (previously called serous cystadenoma). These lesions have no malignant potential.
- Clinical presentation ranges from an asymptomatic, incidental finding to constitutional symptoms of nausea, vomiting, weight loss, and flank or back pain.
- Association with von Hippel-Lindau syndrome has been postulated.
- CT may show a moderately enhancing, well-circumscribed mass anywhere in the pancreas with ovoid or lobular contour, multiple very small cysts, fibrous septa radiating out from a central stellate scar, and occasional punctate calcifications.
- Treatment is surgical resection with serial imaging to verify clinical success.

### ■ Other Imaging Findings

- Ultrasound usually shows an echogenic mass, given the innumerable small cysts, fibrous septations, and tumor cells. Larger cysts may appear hypoechoic.
- Imaging studies show no vascular invasion or encasement, but occasional vascular or ductal compression or displacement.

### ✓ Pearls & ✗ Pitfalls

- ✓ Oligocystic adenoma is an uncommon variant of microcystic adenoma that presents with a few large cysts. Oligocystic adenoma can be indistinguishable from mucinous cystic neoplasm or pseudocyst in some cases.
- ✓ Enhancement on cross-sectional imaging varies among pancreatic tumors, depending on neovascularity, cysts, and central necrosis.
- ✓ In general, pancreatic adenocarcinoma is nonenhancing to minimally enhancing, microcystic adenoma is moderately enhancing, and islet cell tumors are markedly enhancing during the arterial phase.

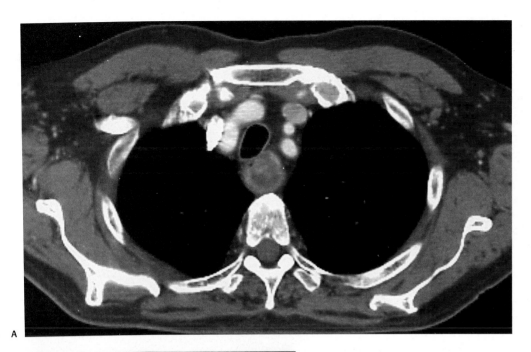

A

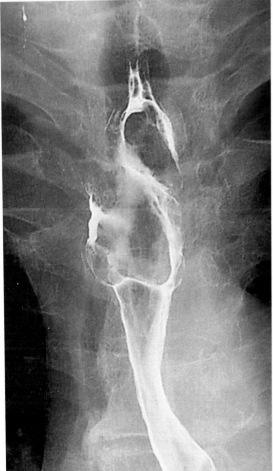

B

### ■ Clinical Presentation

A 62-year-old man presents with dysphagia.

### ■ Imaging Findings

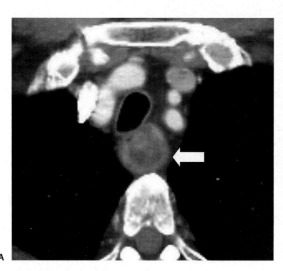

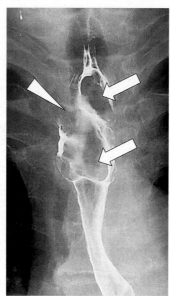

**(A)** Contrast-enhanced computed tomography (CT) shows an upper esophageal soft-tissue mass (*arrow*) with a necrotic center. **(B)** Single-contrast esophagogram shows a large, intraluminal, multilobular polypoid mass (*arrows*). The upper right side of the mass shows a broad, pedunculated attachment to the esophageal wall (*arrowhead*).

### ■ Differential Diagnosis

- **Spindle cell carcinoma:** This is the most likely diagnosis. It is characteristically bulky and polypoid and expands the lumen without complete obstruction, which is consistent with the appearance of this case on the esophagogram.
- *Esophageal carcinoma:* This may present radiologically as a polypoid mass. Adenocarcinoma is more commonly polypoid compared with squamous cell carcinoma, although usually distal.
- *Lymphoma or melanoma:* This may occur anywhere in the esophagus and present as a bulky polypoid mass.

### ■ Essential Facts

- Spindle cell carcinomas are rare malignant tumors formerly called carcinosarcomas because they contain elements of both carcinoma and sarcoma as a result of spindle cell metaplasia. A tendency toward expansion of the lumen without obstruction allows these tumors to become very large before clinical presentation.
- Clinical presentation is similar to that of carcinoma: dysphagia and weight loss.
- Imaging findings: Esophagogram shows a bulky, often multilobulated polypoid mass. CT shows a nonspecific expansile mass.

- Prognosis: same 5-year survival rate (< 10%) as esophageal squamous cell carcinoma or adenocarcinoma, with a similar rate of nodal and hematogenous metastasis and a similar rate of recurrence after resection
- Treatment is radical esophagectomy.
- Adenocarcinoma of the esophagus arises via the dysplasia of gastric epithelial cells, typically within Barrett mucosa (10% risk) and typically in the lower esophagus extending into the stomach.
- Squamous cell carcinoma of the esophagus typically results from smoking or alcohol abuse but may occur with a variety of conditions, such as caustic strictures, celiac disease, and achalasia. It presents more commonly with direct extension to adjacent mediastinal structures despite a prognosis similar to that of spindle cell carcinoma.

### ✓ Pearls & ✗ Pitfalls

- ✓ The differential diagnosis for a polypoid mass in the upper esophagus often includes fibrovascular polyp, but this entity originates in the cervical esophagus, presents as a single, long, smoothly marginated polyp with a thin stalk, and may have areas of fat density detectable on CT.
- ✓ Adenocarcinoma and squamous cell carcinoma may appear as an infiltrative, ulcerated polypoid or varicoid mass.

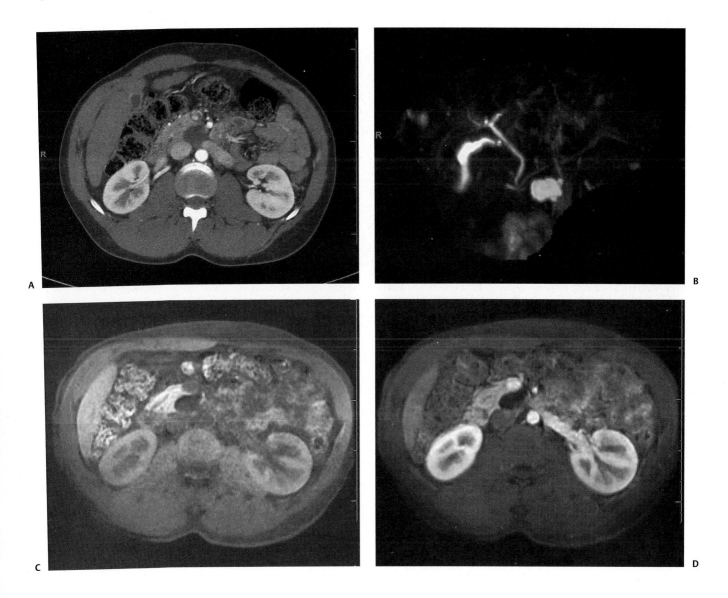

## Clinical Presentation

A 66-year-old man presents with back pain, diarrhea, and fever.

### ◾ Imaging Findings

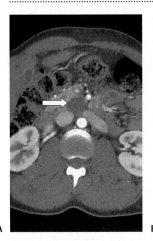
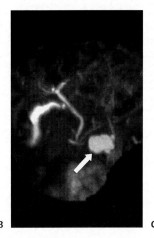
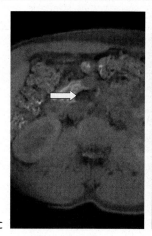
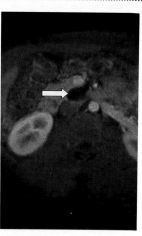

A        B        C        D

**(A)** Contrast-enhanced computed tomography (CT) shows a low-density, well-circumscribed mass (*arrow*) in the uncinate process of the pancreas. **(B)** Magnetic resonance cholangiopancreatography (MRCP) shows the mass (*arrow*) to be communicating with the ventral pancreatic duct and hyperintense on T2. **(C)** Preinfusion T1 image shows the mass (*arrow*) to be hypointense. **(D)** Postinfusion T1 image shows no enhancement (*arrow*).

### ◾ Differential Diagnosis

- ***Intraductal papillary mucinous neoplasm (IPMN):*** This is the first choice for the diagnosis. It most often occurs in men and has a cystic component communicating with a pancreatic duct. The focal type is more common in the pancreatic head. It is distinguished by direct communication of the cyst with the main pancreatic duct or a side branch.
- *Pancreatic pseudocyst:* This is less likely, given that there is no evidence of pancreatitis in the remainder of the pancreatic head.
- *Mucinous cystic neoplasm:* This is less likely and most often occurs in women, usually presenting as a cystic, well-circumscribed mass with enhancing components. It involves the tail in the majority of cases.

### ◾ Essential Facts

- IPMN is a mucin-secreting neoplasm that may involve a main pancreatic duct or a side branch ("branch type") and typically affects older men.
- Clinical presentation is caused by pancreatic duct obstruction and may include diarrhea and back pain, diabetes, and, in cases with superimposed pancreatitis, fever. Transient episodes of pancreatitis may precede the presentation.
- Diffuse IPMN may involve a long segment of the pancreatic duct, causing diffuse ductal dilatation and a papilla that bulges into the duodenum on imaging studies and endoscopy.
- Focal IPMN (branch type or main duct), as in this case, involves a focal segment of duct that dilates to a cystic structure. Communication of this structure with a duct is a characteristic finding, demonstrable by MRCP or endoscopic retrograde cholangiopancreatography.

- Malignant potential is possible for any IPMN and is suggested by:
  - Mass component invading adjacent structures.
  - Enhancing masses or nodules within the cystic lesion or duct.

### ◾ Other Imaging Findings

- CT may demonstrate amorphous calcifications at the periphery of the lesion.

### ✓ Pearls & ✗ Pitfalls

- ✓ Cystic lesions in the pancreas are most commonly pseudocysts (90%) resulting from pancreatitis.
- ✓ Mucinous cystic neoplasm is the main neoplastic differential consideration, but this entity is most commonly larger and multiloculate, with septa and enhancing nodular components.
- ✓ Pancreatic pseudocysts may be indistinguishable from IPMN. Look for evidence of acute or chronic pancreatitis. Imaging findings supporting pancreatitis include the following:
  - Pancreatic enlargement, peripancreatic edema, or fluid
  - Duodenal and gastric wall thickening
  - Low signal intensity on T1-weighted magnetic resonance imaging due to fibrosis
  - Tapered narrowing of the distal common bile duct
- ✗ IPMN may be difficult to distinguish from focal pancreatitis both clinically and on imaging studies.

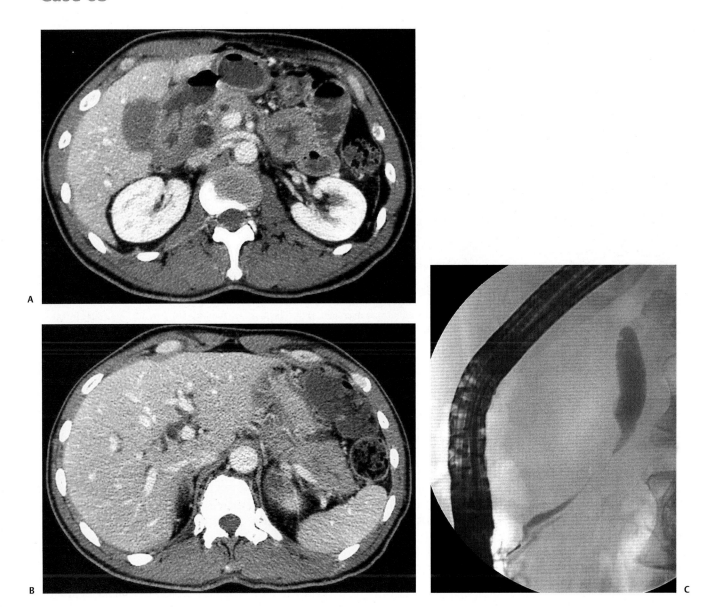

## ▣ Clinical Presentation

A 58-year-old man presents with weight loss and mild right upper quadrant abdominal pain.

## Imaging Findings

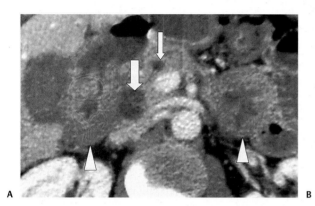
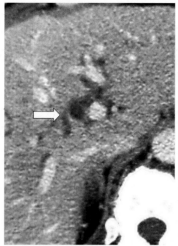
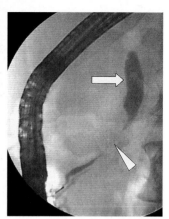

**(A)** Contrast-enhanced computed tomography (CT) shows marked, diffuse thickening of the duodenal wall (*arrowheads*), which is inseparable from the pancreatic head, and dilatation of both the common bile duct (*large arrow*) and the pancreatic duct (*small arrow*). **(B)** Higher cut shows intrahepatic biliary dilatation (*arrow*). **(C)** Endoscopic retrograde cholangiopancreatography shows dilatation of the common bile duct (*large arrow*) with eccentric, shelflike transition to a long, distal stricture (*arrowhead*).

### ■ Differential Diagnosis

- **Duodenal lymphoma:** This infiltrating mass affecting a long segment of small bowel is more likely to be lymphoma than infiltrating adenocarcinoma; hence, it is the first choice for the correct diagnosis.
- *Metastatic disease:* This may have a variety of appearances, but it is more commonly located in the jejunum. It is usually melanoma and less commonly breast, lung, gastrointestinal, or genitourinary primaries.
- *Primary adenocarcinoma:* This is the statistically less likely option for the diagnosis; although similar to lymphoma, a primary adenocarcinoma may be an infiltrative or focal polypoid mass that may ulcerate.

### ■ Essential Facts

- Lymphoma is the most common small-bowel malignancy. It usually involves other locations before affecting the small bowel, and other portions of the small bowel more commonly than the duodenum (ileum > jejunum). Non-Hodgkin lymphoma of the small bowel is much more common than Hodgkin lymphoma.
- Small-bowel lymphoma can be primary or secondary to a predisposing condition.
- Predisposing conditions include celiac disease, Crohn disease, human immunodeficiency virus infection, other causes of immune compromise, and Middle Eastern descent.
- On imaging studies, duodenal lymphoma can have a variety of appearances, including subtle thickening and disruption of the fold pattern, wall thickening, focal polypoid mass(es), an ulcerating or cavitary mass, and infiltration of a long segment of small bowel.

- Infiltration of a long segment, as in this case, is the most common pattern seen in the small bowel and often results in decreased or absent peristalsis and aneurysmal dilatation, rather than stricture of the affected segment, due to disruption of the autonomic plexus. This finding may be associated with the absence of small-bowel obstruction.
- If the autonomic plexus is intact, infiltration typically results in stricture formation with bowel obstruction.

### ■ Other Imaging Findings

- CT typically shows larger mesenteric lymph nodes in small-bowel lymphoma compared with the lymphadenopathy associated with other small-bowel malignancies. Normal abdominal lymph nodes are ≤ 11 mm.
- Lymph nodes may appear as a large confluent mass encasing other structures.

### ✓ Pearls & ✗ Pitfalls

- ✓ Lymphoma may involve the stomach and duodenum by crossing the pylorus, may involve the biliary system, and may result in fistulae to other bowel loops.
- ✓ Intussusception is common in small-bowel lymphoma occurring in children but may also be seen in adults. Ileal lymphoma is particularly prone to ileocolic intussusception.
- ✓ Malabsorption is occasionally associated with diffuse lymphoma of the small bowel.
- ✗ Do not miss perforation, which often occurs with lymphoma that is ulcerated or being treated with chemotherapy!

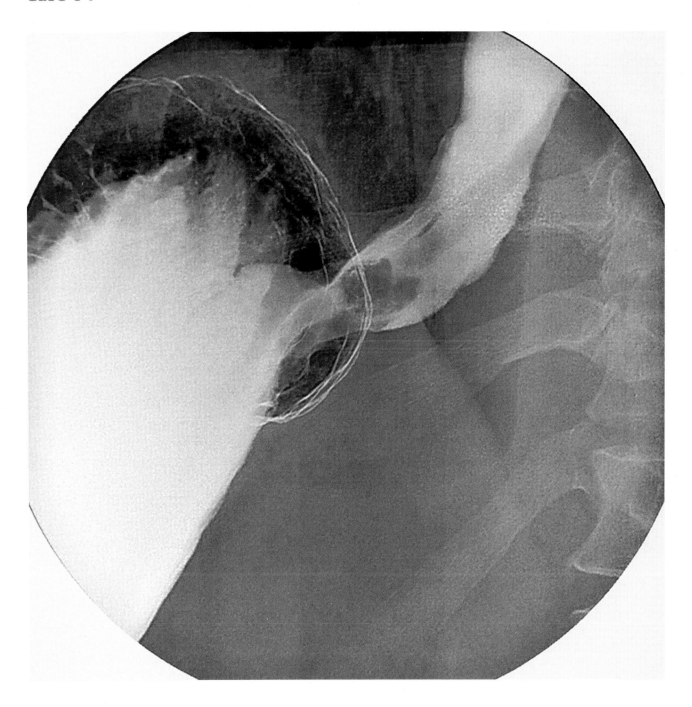

## Clinical Presentation

A 51-year-old man presents with a history of gastroesophageal reflux.

### ▇ Imaging Findings

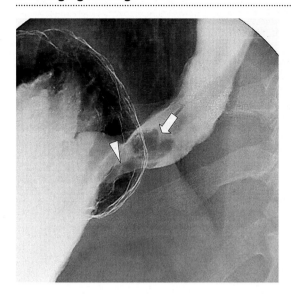

Single-contrast barium swallow shows a bilobed polyp (*arrow*) in the distal esophagus arising near the esophagogastric junction. The polyp appears pedunculated and continues from a prominent gastric fold (*arrowhead*).

### ▇ Differential Diagnosis

- ***Inflammatory esophagogastric polyp:*** This is the top choice for the diagnosis and is associated with reflux esophagitis, presented in this patient's history. The findings in this case are quite characteristic.
- *Inflammatory myofibroblastic pseudotumors:* This is a remote possibility and may also arise near the esophagogastric junction.
- *Gastric adenocarcinoma:* This can be polypoid and occur at this location. Nodularity, irregular contour, or ulceration would raise suspicion for malignancy, but these are not present in this case.

### ▇ Essential Facts

- The key to this case is having a good differential for intramural polypoid lesions of the esophagus and the ability to rank lesions based on location.
- Inflammatory esophagogastric polyp originates from the gastric side of the squamocolumnar junction and may be a localized form of hypertrophic gastritis.
  - Associated with reflux esophagitis, hiatal hernias, and Barrett esophagus; postulated to be localized hypertrophic gastritis
  - Histopathology is hyperplastic epithelium with variable amounts of inflamed stroma.

- Imaging findings include a smoothly marginated polyp near the squamocolumnar junction that appears to be a continuation of a linear gastric fold.
- Inflammatory myofibroblastic pseudotumor is a polyp arising from the mucosa and containing granulation tissue and bizarre stromal cells (likely neoplastic rather than hyperplastic).
  - Viral associations proposed: Epstein-Barr virus, human papillomavirus, herpesvirus
- Fibrovascular polyps are composed of connective tissue, adipose tissue, and vascular structures and are covered by squamous epithelium.
  - Usually in the cervical esophagus, they may be large and pedunculated and rarely cause asphyxiation by regurgitation and impaction at the glottis.

### ✓ Pearls & ✗ Pitfalls

- ✓ Ulceration, mural irregularity, nodularity, and significant luminal attenuation are worrisome for malignancy and should prompt endoscopy.
- ✗ Carcinoma can masquerade as benign lesions and present at any level of the esophagus as a smoothly marginated mucosal lesion or polyp.

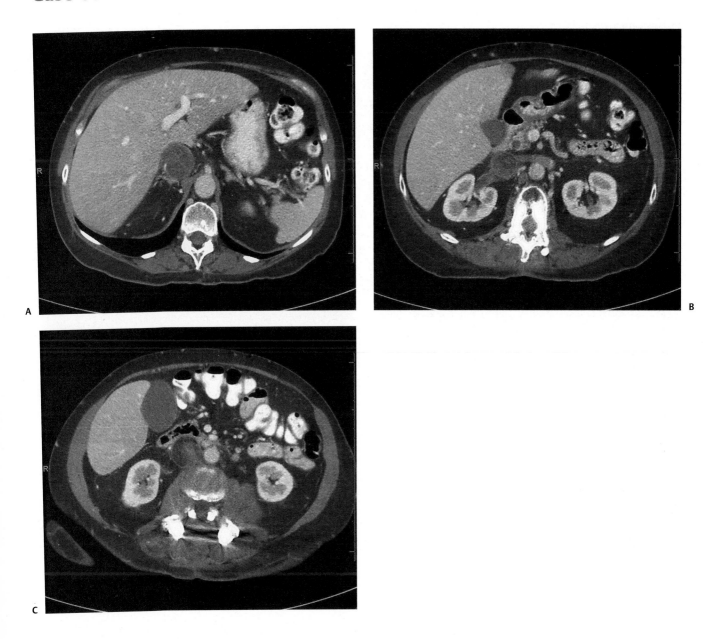

A

B

C

## Clinical Presentation

A 50-year-old woman presents with back pain, nausea, and weight loss.

## ▇ Imaging Findings

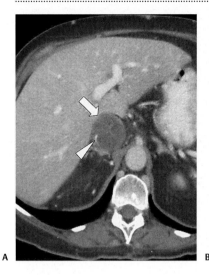 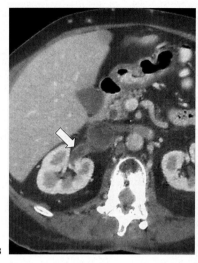 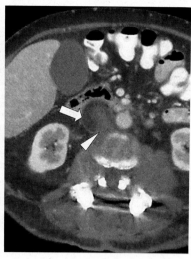

**(A)** Contrast-enhanced computed tomography (CT) shows marked enlargement of the inferior vena cava (IVC; *arrow*) with obliteration of the lumen by soft tissue. Arterial branches (*arrowhead*) course through this soft tissue. **(B)** More caudal image shows extension of the mass into the right renal vein (*arrow*). The mass appears more heterogeneous in density at this level. The kidney parenchyma is normal. **(C)** More caudal image shows a fatty component (*arrow*) of the intraluminal IVC mass, which extends outside the confines of the IVC into the retroperitoneal fat (*arrowhead*).

## ▇ Differential Diagnosis

- ***Liposarcoma locally invasive to the IVC:*** This is the most likely explanation for a vascular soft-tissue mass with a component of macroscopic fat occurring within the retroperitoneum, albeit within the IVC itself.
- *Malignant teratoma:* This is a second possibility that may have fat and soft-tissue components, but the more typical toothlike calcifications are absent in this case.

## ▇ Essential Facts

- The key to this case is recognizing the difference between malignant tumor and thrombus (see "Pearls & Pitfalls") within the IVC and then successfully characterizing this mass as a liposarcoma based on local invasion and fat content.
- Liposarcoma is a tumor of mesenchymal origin that usually presents in middle age. It is more common in women. Liposarcoma is the most common primary retroperitoneal neoplasm.
- Locations: liposarcoma typically occurs in the mesentery, omentum, and retroperitoneum, particularly behind the kidney.
- CT findings:
  - Heterogeneous masses with fat and soft tissue should prompt consideration of liposarcoma.
  - Fat is almost always present in liposarcomas and absent in other soft-tissue sarcomas, such as malignant fibrous histiocytoma and leiomyosarcoma.

- Mass effect often predominates over local invasion of adjacent structures.
- Liposarcomas are quite large at presentation in most cases.
- Prognosis: 5-year survival rate is 30 to 40%.

## ✓ Pearls & ✗ Pitfalls

- ✓ Tumor thrombus within the IVC is actually intraluminal growth of tumor.
- ✓ Tumor thrombus often enhances and is often associated with an adjacent tumor.
- ✓ Growth is often slow enough that symptoms of IVC obstruction associated with bland thrombus do not occur.
- ✓ Malignancies can be secondary, invading the IVC from the retroperitoneum or extending from organs that drain into the IVC. Such neoplasms include adrenal, renal cell, and hepatocellular carcinomas.
- ✓ Malignancies arising from the IVC itself are rarely primary; the most common primary malignancy of the IVC is leiomyosarcoma, which is the top consideration for an intraluminal tumor if no adjacent masses are present.
- ✗ Malignant tumors of the mesentery may surround mesenteric fat and create the appearance of fat components within a teratoma or liposarcoma.
- ✗ Tumor thrombus and bland thrombus often coexist. Look for foci of enhancement or local invasion!

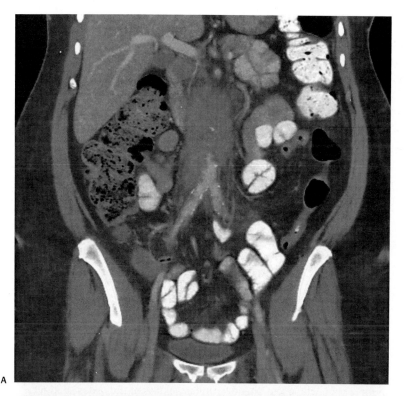

A

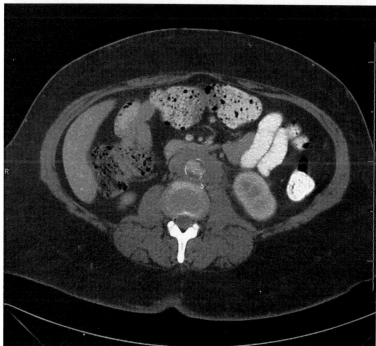

B

## Clinical Presentation

A 69-year-old woman presents with flank pain.

■ **Imaging Findings**

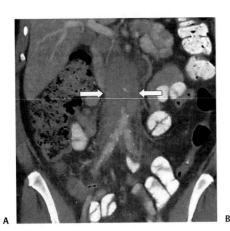 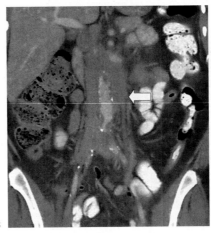 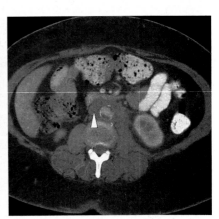

A　　　　　　　　　　　B　　　　　　　　　　　C

**(A)** Coronal reformatted infused computed tomography (CT) image shows a soft-tissue mass (*arrows*) encasing the inferior vena cava and aorta. **(B)** Adjacent image shows the mass encasing the left ureter (*arrow*). **(C)** Axial image shows the mass (*arrowhead*) enveloping the aorta and displacing the inferior vena cava. No vascular invasion is apparent.

■ **Differential Diagnosis**

- **Retroperitoneal fibrosis:** This is the most likely diagnosis for soft-tissue infiltration of the retroperitoneum encasing, but not invading or displacing, retroperitoneal structures.
- *Retroperitoneal soft-tissue tumors:* These are often aggressive and invade rather than encase. Here, the proliferating fibrous connective tissue appears masslike, and any retroperitoneal soft-tissue sarcoma is a consideration.

■ **Essential Facts**

- Retroperitoneal fibrosis is the extensive proliferation of fibrous connective tissue within the retroperitoneum.
- In this case, the masslike appearance raises the question of a soft-tissue sarcoma. The absence of local invasion or marked displacement of adjacent structures and the absence of distant metastasis to liver or lung argue against sarcomas.
- Retroperitoneal fibrosis is most commonly idiopathic but is postulated to be immune-mediated. Retroperitoneal surgery, tumor, infection, inflammation, bleeding, and the migraine medication methysergide have been postulated as possible causes.
- Associations include immune-mediated disorders such as rheumatoid arthritis, systemic lupus erythematosus, polyarteritis nodosa, and ankylosing spondylitis.
- Retroperitoneal fibrosis may continue across the diaphragm as or occur with mediastinal fibrosis.
- CT may show soft tissue surrounding the aorta, inferior vena cava, renal veins, and ureters with no clear fat plane between the soft tissue and the psoas muscle.
- Treatment is surgical lysis of the fibrous tissue causing symptoms (gold standard). Steroids and immunosuppressive drugs have been used adjunctively.

■ **Other Imaging Findings**

- Abdominal radiography may show bilateral loss of the psoas shadow. Unilateral loss of the psoas shadow is more consistent with retroperitoneal masses and abscesses.

✓ **Pearls &** ✗ **Pitfalls**

- ✓ Soft-tissue sarcomas occurring in the retroperitoneum tend to be large and malignant, including (in order of frequency) liposarcoma > leiomyosarcoma > malignant fibrous histiocytoma.
  - Unlike retroperitoneal sarcomas, retroperitoneal fibrosis encases structures without invading or displacing them.
  - Like retroperitoneal sarcomas, retroperitoneal fibrosis can appear masslike.
- ✗ Soft-tissue sarcomas rarely metastasize to lymph nodes. Therefore, the absence of lymphadenopathy does not distinguish these entities from retroperitoneal fibrosis.

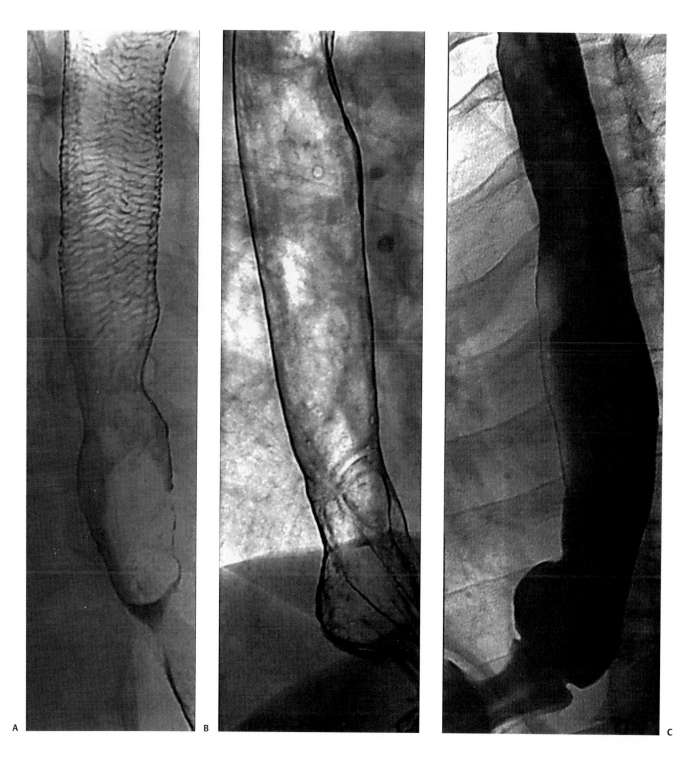

A          B          C

## ■ Clinical Presentation

Three different men in their mid-30s present with dysphagia and chest pain. What is the clinical significance of each diagnosis?

### ■ Imaging Findings

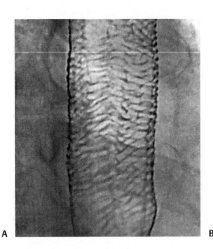 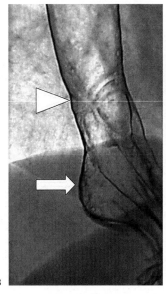 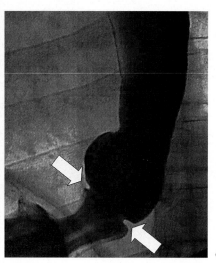

**(A)** Double-contrast esophagogram shows a lattice of horizontal lines throughout the esophageal mucosa, indicating feline esophagus. **(B)** Double-contrast esophagogram shows a focus of transverse lines (*arrowhead*) a few centimeters above the gastroesophageal junction, indicating a peptic stricture from reflux esophagitis and a small hiatal hernia (*arrow*). **(C)** Single-contrast esophagogram shows a narrow horizontal ring (*arrows*) at the distal esophagus just above a small hiatal hernia, indicating a B ring.

### ■ Differential Diagnosis

- **Benign transverse esophageal folds:** No differential diagnosis is necessary because a single diagnosis can be assigned to each case based on classic imaging findings.

### ■ Essential Facts

- This case illustrates the importance of recognizing and identifying benign transverse rings, lines, and folds seen on esophagogram. Clinical significance depends on the type of line identified.
- Feline esophagus:
  - Transient diffuse contraction of the longitudinal muscularis mucosae causes thin transverse folds in a diffuse, regular pattern that spans the width of the esophagus.
  - Feline esophagus is asymptomatic but may be an indicator of gastroesophageal reflux.
- Peptic strictures:
  - These are typically distal, smoothly marginated, and concentric, although asymmetric scarring may cause eccentric narrowing.
  - Longitudinal scarring and contraction cause fixed transverse folds, like the ones in Figure B, that are thicker than those of feline esophagus and fail to traverse the entire width of the esophagus.
- B ring or Schatzki ring:
  - This is a smooth, abruptly marginated, symmetric ring measuring < 3 mm in thickness and occurring at the esophagogastric junction just below the mucosal junction (squamocolumnar junction or Z line).

- B rings are seen only when drawn craniad by the presence of a hiatal hernia and are best visualized with the esophagus fully distended.

### ✓ Pearls & ✗ Pitfalls

- ✓ Esophageal strictures are typically clinical significant if they fail to allow passage of a 12-mm-diameter barium tablet.
- ✓ Focal peptic strictures can be mistaken for Schatzki rings but are typically thicker (> 4 mm) and asymmetrical, with smoother, tapering margination. Both can occur at the gastroesophageal junction, with clinical implications.
- ✓ Schatzki rings may progress to distal esophageal strictures in the setting of reflux esophagitis, although this spectrum is somewhat controversial.
- ✓ The Z line is a more subtle line indicating the squamocolumnar mucosal junction, which is just above the gastroesophageal junction. Other than the presence of Barrett mucosa above this line, it has no clinical significance.
- ✓ Esophageal webs usually occur in the cervical esophagus but may occur elsewhere. A relationship with gastroesophageal reflux has been suggested for some webs.

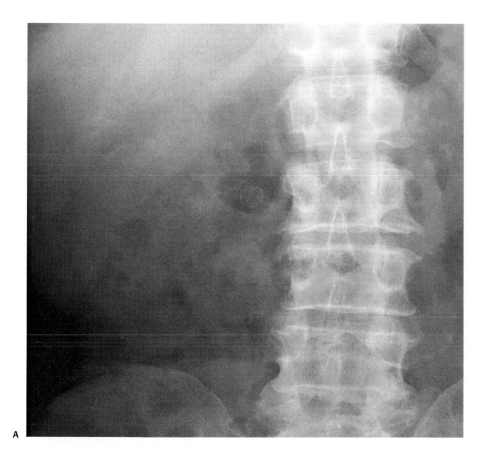

A

## Clinical Presentation

A 68-year-old man presents for the evaluation of right upper quadrant pain.

## Further Work-up

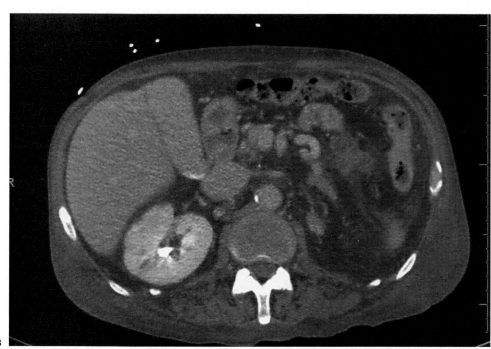

B

■ **Imaging Findings**

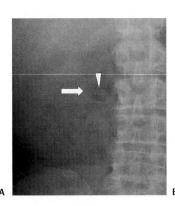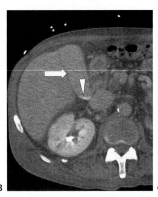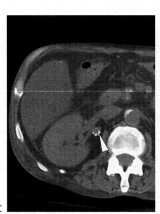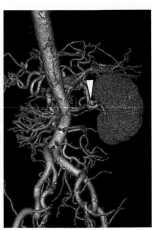

A · B · C · D

**(A)** Frontal abdominal radiograph shows a gas-filled structure in the right upper quadrant (*arrow*) superimposed on a small, round, calcified structure (*arrowhead*). **(B)** Contrast-enhanced computed tomography (CT) shows the gallbladder (*arrow*) to be fluid-filled (not gas-filled), with small, layering stones (*arrowhead*) but no large, calcified gallstones. **(C)** Noninfused CT shows a rounded, calcified structure adjacent to the renal artery (*arrowhead*). **(D)** CT angiography verifies renal artery aneurysm (*arrowhead*).

■ **Differential Diagnosis**

• ***Aneurysm:*** This is the most likely diagnosis. Here, an aneurysm of the renal, hepatic, or gastroduodenal artery and branches should be considered for a round, calcified structure in the right upper quadrant. This case is made more difficult by superimposed duodenal bowel gas.
• *Emphysematous cholecystitis:* At first glance, this is the choice diagnosis based on radiographic findings suggesting a gallstone within a gas-filled gallbladder. However, the clinical presentation would be grave, and the CT findings are inconsistent with this diagnosis.
• *Calcified lymphadenopathy within the porta hepatis or mesentery:* This may be suggested by this radiographic appearance.

■ **Essential Facts**

• The differential diagnosis for this case is tricky because of a rounded, calcified structure superimposed on a rounded, gas-filled structure.
• Curvilinear or rounded calcifications in the right upper quadrant on abdominal radiographs are nonspecific and should be initially addressed with a broad differential diagnosis, including aneurysm, pseudoaneurysm, stone (renal, biliary, or cholecystic), cyst (mesenteric, enteric duplication, pancreatic, renal, or hepatic), or mass.
• Round, air-filled structures in the right upper quadrant may be emphysematous cholecystitis, emphysematous pyonephrosis, gas-containing abscess, gas within a bowel loop, or loculate free air.

• Less likely diagnostic alternatives:
  • Emphysematous pyonephrosis, which is obstruction of the ureteropelvic junction caused by a stone, is also a viable option for the radiographic findings, but not for the clinical presentation or CT findings.
  • Calcified mass involving the pancreas, kidney, bowel, mesentery, or abdominal wall also may have this radiographic appearance.

■ **Other Imaging Findings**

• On CT, hypodense, rounded structures in the abdomen may represent saccular aneurysms or pseudoaneurysms. Distinction is critical as biopsy, needle aspiration, or tube drainage may be planned. Consider a Doppler study or infused CT before recommending intervention.

✓ **Pearls & ✗ Pitfalls**

✓ Separate the radiographic findings to provide a differential diagnosis for each.
✓ Consider the clinical information and start with a broad differential including all organ systems in the region of each abnormality.
✗ This case illustrates the danger of associating multiple radiographic findings to assign a single diagnosis (emphysematous cholecystitis).

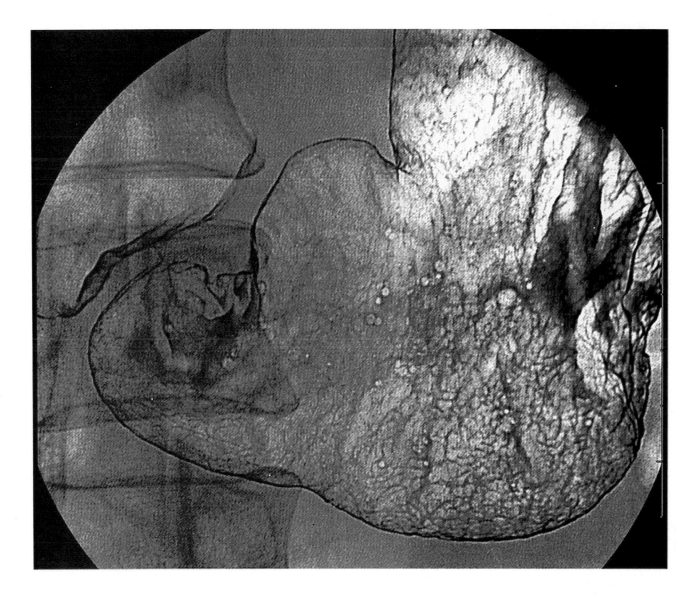

## Clinical Presentation

A 43-year-old man presents with substernal pressure and burning.

## ▣ Imaging Findings

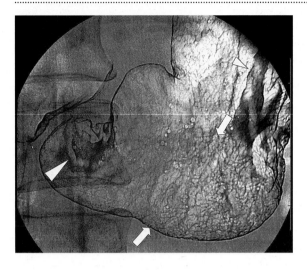

Double-contrast upper gastrointestinal study shows diffuse enlargement of the areae gastricae (*arrows*) with a polygonal shape and thickening of the rugal folds of the gastric body (*small arrowhead*) and antrum (*large arrowhead*).

## ▣ Differential Diagnosis

- **Hypertrophic gastritis:** This is the most likely diagnosis for enlarged areae gastricae and thickened rugal folds, as well as the clinical history of substernal burning.
- *Antral gastritis:* This is an option as acute gastritis and is included here because it causes thickened rugal folds, particularly along the lesser curvature, as seen in this case. Antral gastritis is limited radiographically to the antrum, but endoscopy often shows more diffuse gastric involvement.
- *Eosinophilic gastritis:* This can cause rugal fold thickening but typically resolves with steroids.

## ▣ Essential Facts

- Hypertrophic gastritis is hyperplasia of the gastric glandular epithelium, thought to be caused by chronic inflammation.
- Glandular epithelial hyperplasia can lead to hypersecretion of gastrin and acid, resulting in Zollinger-Ellison syndrome. Look for resultant superimposed acute gastritis and peptic ulcer disease.
- Barium studies show pleomorphic, enlarged areae gastricae (3–5 mm in diameter) as a sign of chronic hypertrophic gastritis and thickened rugal folds as a sign of superimposed acute gastritis. The areae gastricae are normally 1 to 2 mm and ovoid.
- Infection with *Helicobacter pylori*, a Gram-negative bacillus, commonly causes hypertrophic gastritis. Features include the following:
  - Prominent areae gastricae
  - Gastric fold thickening that is often striking
  - Increased risk for adenocarcinoma and lymphoma
  - Increased risk for gastric and duodenal ulcers
- Diagnosis is made by endoscopic biopsy or serologic testing.

## ▣ Other Imaging Findings

- Look carefully for an ulcer in the stomach or duodenum whenever enlarged areae gastricae are demonstrated.

## ✓ Pearls & ✗ Pitfalls

- ✓ Ménétrier disease can cause rugal fold thickening due to foveolar rather than glandular epithelial hyperplasia. This entity typically spares the antrum and was therefore left off the differential in this case.
- ✓ Lymphoma can cause the focal thickening of the rugal folds seen in this case.
- ✗ Hypertrophic gastritis is a controversial entity of unclear etiology and clinical significance.

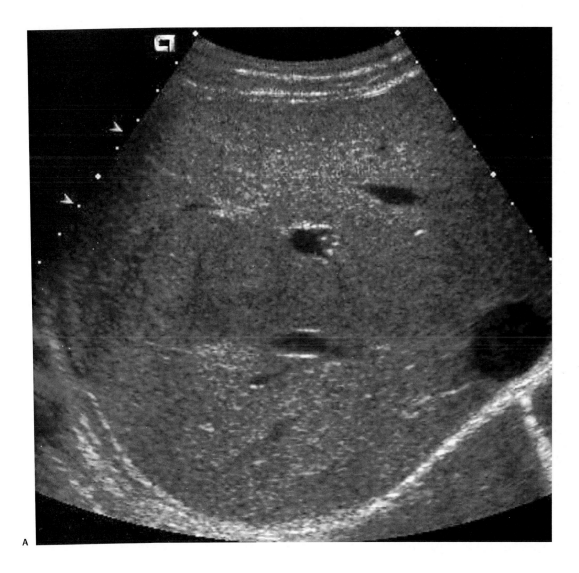

A

## Clinical Presentation

A 35-year-old woman presents with vague right upper quadrant pain.

## Further Work-up

Describe this follow-up study and amend the differential diagnosis if necessary.

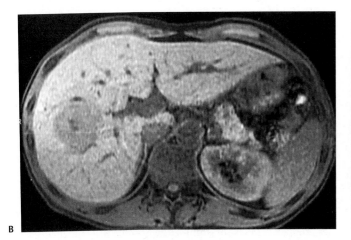

B

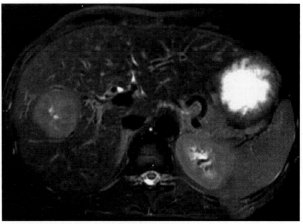

C

### ■ Imaging Findings

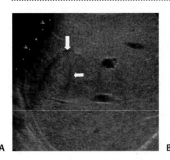 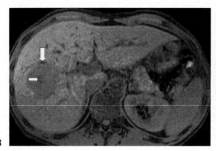 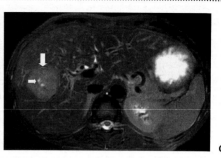

**(A)** Transverse ultrasound shows a well-circumscribed lesion (*large arrow*) that is slightly hypoechoic to liver with a hypoechoic center (*small arrow*). **(B,C)** T1 (B) and T2 fat saturation (C) axial magnetic resonance imaging (MRI): the lesion is slightly hypointense to liver on T1 with a hypointense center and hyperintense to liver on T2 (*large arrows*) with a hyperintense center (*small arrows*).

### ■ Differential Diagnosis

- **Focal nodular hyperplasia (FNH):** In a young woman, a lesion that is slightly hypointense on T1 and slightly hyperintense on T2 with a very hyperintense central scar is most likely FNH.
- *Adenoma:* This is second because of the high incidence and variable appearance. It may be hyperintense on T1, rather than hypointense like FNH, because of fat and glycogen. The vascular supply of adenoma is often draped at periphery, not in central scar as in FNH.
- *Fibrolamellar hepatoma:* This is uncommon but may have a central scar and occur in young patients without cirrhosis.

### ■ Essential Facts

- On ultrasound, a well-defined mass with a central scar is nonspecific. In addition to the items in this differential, metastases, cholangiocarcinoma, and hemangioma may have this appearance.
- FNH is the second most common benign hepatic tumor (after hemangioma).
  - Histology is disorganized, non-neoplastic liver tissue with central arteries ("scar") and no portal supply.
  - Presentation is usually in younger women (20–40 years of age), but it can occur at any age. It is rare in men. It is asymptomatic until growth causes pain.
  - FNH has an association (small) with hemangiomas, intracranial berry aneurysms, and sickle cell anemia, *not* with oral contraceptives (unlike adenoma).
  - Small (3 cm) and solitary at average presentation; necrosis, hemorrhage, and rupture are uncommon.
  - FNH is usually sulfur colloid–positive (has Kupffer cells).
- Adenoma:
  - Most result from oral contraceptive use; they are associated with glycogen storage disease.
  - Benign, mostly hepatocytes (sometimes fatty); necrosis, hemorrhage, and rupture are common.
  - Adenoma is large (9 cm) and solitary at average presentation.
- Fibrolamellar carcinoma:
  - Slow-growing with a better prognosis than hepatoma

- Usually affects younger patients (before 40 years of age) without cirrhosis
- Usually presents with pain and weight loss

### ■ Other Imaging Findings

- Technetium-99m sulfur colloid study: FNH ranges from cold to hot; normal to hot uptake in 70% distinguishes FNH from adenoma (usually cold).
- Computed tomography (CT): without contrast, FNH is homogeneous and hypodense with a hypodense scar (seen in one-third of cases); it enhances in arterial phase but may be isodense in portal phase (often missed on portal-phase CT).
- MRI (best study): Without contrast, FNH is usually isointense on T1 and slightly hyperintense on T2; scar is hypointense on T1 and hyperintense on T2. FNH enhances in arterial phase with delayed enhancement of scar.

### ✓ Pearls & ✗ Pitfalls

✓ Compared with adenoma, FNH more commonly has scar, rarely ruptures, and is not associated with oral contraceptives. Adenoma may drop signal intensity on out-of-phase gradient-echo images because of fatty hepatocytes and glycogen.

✓ Compared with fibrolamellar hepatoma, FNH is more often asymptomatic, its scar rarely calcifies (vs. up to half of fibrolamellar hepatomas), and its scar is hyperintense on T2 (fibrolamellar hepatoma is usually hypointense). FNH enhances homogeneously in arterial phase; fibrolamellar hepatoma enhances heterogeneously in the arterial and portal phases.

✗ Central scar is nonspecific, occurring in only 50% of cases of FNH and also with fibrolamellar hepatomas and adenomas (central hemorrhage).

✗ FNH may be missed on ultrasound, noninfused CT, or delayed contrast-enhanced CT (often looks like normal liver).

✗ FNH and adenoma may enhance early on MRI and CT, washing out on delayed imaging.

✗ FNH and fibrolamellar hepatoma may have a hyperintense scar on T2 (fibrolamellar usually hypointense).

✗ Biopsy is necessary if imaging findings are equivocal.

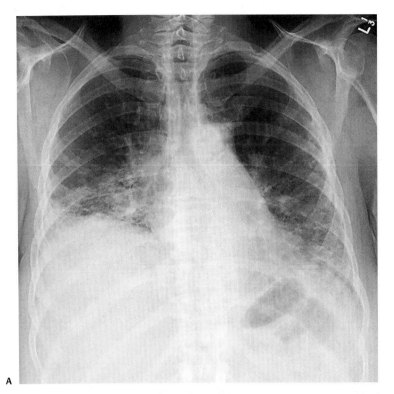

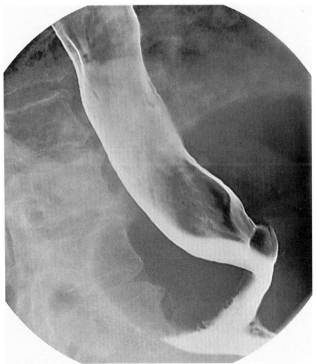

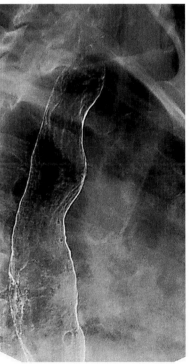

A

B

C

## ■ Clinical Presentation

A 68-year-old woman has gastroesophageal reflux and midepigastric pain.

### ◼ Imaging Findings

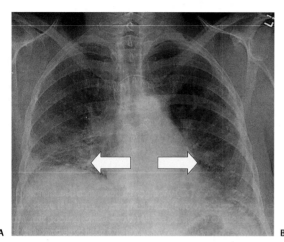
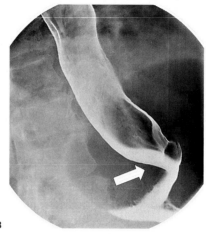
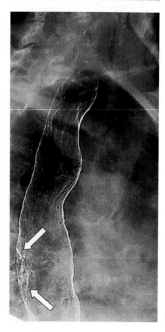

**(A)** Frontal chest radiograph shows bilateral basilar interstitial lung disease (*arrows*). **(B)** Upright barium esophagogram shows a widely patent gastroesophageal junction (*arrow*). **(C)** A focal segment of the dorsum of the esophagus shows mucosal irregularity (*arrows*), possibly representing esophagitis.

### ◼ Differential Diagnosis

- **Scleroderma:** This is the most likely diagnosis, given the patulous esophagus and the bilateral basilar interstitial lung disease.
- *Rheumatoid arthritis:* This is a possibility as it can result in an atonic esophagus and interstitial lung disease.
- *Systemic lupus erythematosus, polymyositis/dermatomyositis:* This, as well as anticholinergic medications, can cause an atonic esophagus, simulating scleroderma.

### ◼ Essential Facts

- Scleroderma involves the gastrointestinal tract in 90% and the esophagus in 80%.
- Clinical presentation is usually retention of food and debris in the esophagus due to decreased peristalsis; retention is particularly prominent in the supine position. The patulous gastroesophageal junction and dysmotility cause reflux, which may result in strictures or esophagitis (in 40%).
- Pathogenesis is atrophy of smooth muscle, then fibrosis and collagen deposition.
- Because the upper third of the esophagus is striated muscle and the lower two-thirds is smooth muscle, the primary wave may clear the upper one-third but terminate abruptly at the level of the aortic arch.
- Radiograph may show bilateral basilar interstitial lung disease and an air-filled esophagus, as in this case.

### ◼ Other Imaging Findings

- Esophagography is best performed with the patient supine, which emphasizes retention of barium in an atonic esophagus.
  - Motility: interruption of the peristaltic wave, diminished peristalsis, gastroesophageal reflux
  - Other findings: esophagitis (as in this case), Barrett esophagus, peptic strictures, esophageal dilatation, and esophageal carcinoma

### ✓ Pearls & ✗ Pitfalls

- ✓ Both achalasia and scleroderma may manifest with esophageal retention and dilatation.
  - Unlike patients with achalasia, those with scleroderma empty the esophagus by gravity through a patulous esophagus when placed upright.
  - Patients with achalasia have beaklike narrowing of the distal esophagus rather than a patulous gastroesophageal junction.
- ✓ The differential diagnosis for esophageal scleroderma includes any diseases causing atony and dilatation.
- ✗ Esophagography in the upright position may miss the interruption of the peristaltic wave associated with scleroderma.

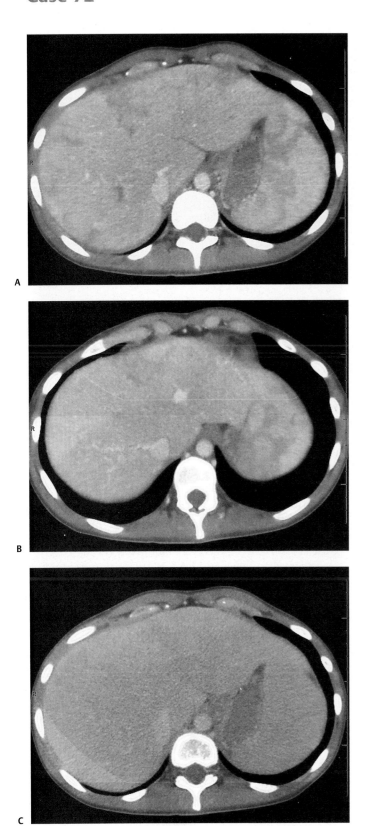

A

B

C

## Clinical Presentation

A 23-year-old woman presents with abdominal distension.

## Imaging Findings

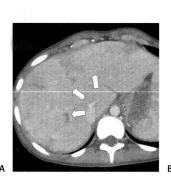 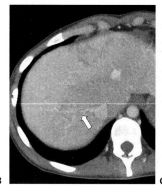 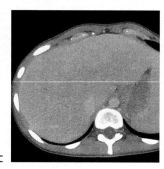 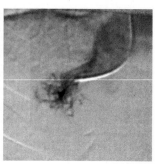

A           B           C           D

**(A)** Contrast-enhanced computed tomography (CT) shows heterogeneous peripheral enhancement (*arrows*), homogeneous central enhancement, and left lobe hypertrophy. **(B)** The right hepatic vein (*arrow*) appears occluded. **(C)** Delayed image shows homogeneous enhancement of the entire liver. **(D)** Transjugular hepatic venography shows the "spiderweb" pattern of hepatic veins, consistent with Budd-Chiari syndrome.

## Differential Diagnosis

- **Budd-Chiari syndrome (BCS):** This is the top choice for the diagnosis as it classically presents with delayed peripheral hepatic enhancement. This is further supported by the tortuous, narrowed right hepatic vein in Figure B.
- *Cirrhosis (without BCS):* This can result in relative sparing of the left lobe, mottled enhancement, and tortuous vessels in the liver ("corkscrew" hepatic arteries).
- *Right heart failure:* This may result in hepatic venous congestion and mottled, delayed enhancement. Hepatic veins are often congested rather than fibrosed, as in this case.

## Essential Facts

- BCS is acute or chronic obstruction of the venous outflow of the liver, which may result from obstruction of the hepatic veins, inferior vena cava (IVC), or both.
  - Acute: collateral venous channels to the IVC have not fully developed, and symptoms develop more rapidly, including nausea, vomiting, and abdominal distention from marked ascites.
  - Subacute: Collaterals partially develop before symptoms become severe. Ascites may be minimal.
  - Chronic: presenting features are those of cirrhosis and portal hypertension, such as variceal bleeding.
- Causes include hypercoagulable states, myeloproliferative disorders, oral contraceptives, pregnancy, venous webs, infection, and tumor infiltration or compression.
- Treatment:
  - Medical options may be sufficient for mild cases, including correction of coagulopathy and management of ascites with diuretics and paracentesis.
  - Endovascular options include catheter-directed thrombolysis for acute thrombosis, angioplasty for stenoses or webs, and transjugular intrahepatic portosystemic stent-shunt for chronic BCS with esophagogastric variceal bleeding or refractory ascites.

- Surgical options include mesocaval or splenorenal shunt and transplantation, but these options are reserved for refractory cases.

## Other Imaging Findings

- Common imaging findings include early hepatomegaly and ascites, and later left lobe and caudate enlargement (separate venous drainage to the IVC). Hepatic veins may be thrombosed, small, or difficult to see.
- CT and magnetic resonance imaging may show early heterogeneous and delayed homogeneous peripheral enhancement due to delayed transit of contrast through the sinusoids.
- Ultrasound may show direct or indirect evidence of obstructed outflow veins, such as webs, thrombus, stenosis, nonvisualized hepatic veins, and slow, reversed, or bidirectional hepatic or portal venous flow.
- Venography may show spiderweb collaterals in addition to the venous abnormalities previously listed.

## ✓ Pearls & ✗ Pitfalls

- ✓ Infection, inflammation, or neoplastic infiltration can cause mottling of liver enhancement and focal areas of hypertrophy.
- ✓ Hepatic veno-occlusive disease is considered a separate entity by most authors.
  - Obstruction of the hepatic venules results from inflammation and fibrosis, typically after high-dose chemotherapy and hematopoietic stem cell transplant.
- ✗ Hepatic veno-occlusive disease may mimic graft-versus-host disease clinically and is usually associated with patent hepatic veins and IVC. Biopsy is typically required.

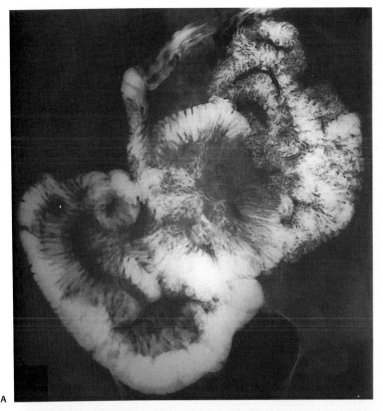

A

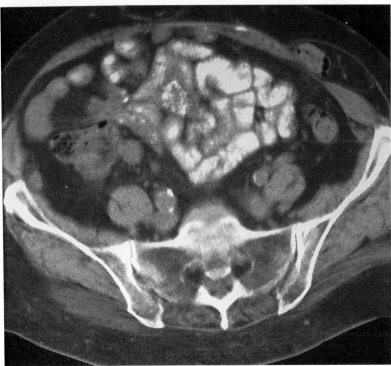

B

## ▓ Clinical Presentation

A 45-year-old man presents with intermittent watery diarrhea.

## ■ Imaging Findings

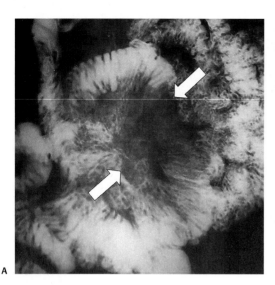
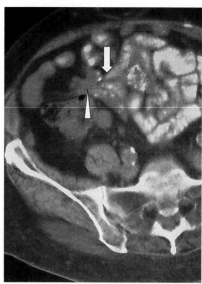

**(A)** Barium small-bowel series shows a group of separated jejunal loops (*arrows*) that appear to be tethered at the center. **(B)** Noninfused computed tomography (CT) shows a spicular, partially calcified mesenteric soft-tissue mass (*arrowhead*) with associated tethering of adjacent small bowel (*arrow*).

## ■ Differential Diagnosis

- **Small-bowel mesenteric carcinoid:** A spiculated, calcified mass at the mesenteric root, tethered small bowel, and watery diarrhea are highly suggestive of this entity.
- *Retractile mesenteritis:* This is a classic alternative to carcinoid for soft-tissue thickening centered at the superior mesenteric root. The calcifications are typically denser than those of carcinoid.
- *Metastatic disease:* A desmoplastic reaction may occur with primary malignancies of the pancreas, ovary, and breast.

## ■ Essential Facts

- Carcinoid is an uncommon, slow-growing neoplasm with variable malignant potential arising from a variety of neuroendocrine cell types.
- Location is the gastrointestinal (GI) tract in > 90%, and the midgut from the distal duodenum to the proximal transverse colon in 80%.
- Appearance in the small bowel depends largely on the point of diagnosis:
  - Early small-bowel carcinoids are mucosal or submucosal, well defined, and similar in appearance to lipoma, adenoma, lymphoma, leiomyoma, or metastases.
  - Later small-bowel carcinoids may ulcerate, producing a bull's-eye appearance similar to that of Kaposi sarcoma, lymphoma, or metastases from melanoma or breast carcinoma.
- Infiltrating small-bowel carcinoids grow into the bowel wall, lymphatics, and mesentery, leading to the desmoplastic reaction.

- Desmoplastic reaction is the release of vasoactive substances (e.g., peptides, serotonin) that cause mesenteric fibrosis.
- Small-bowel series may show a smooth, submucosal mass with bowel wall and fold thickening progressing to fixed, angulated, narrowed, and/or kinked small-bowel loops.
- CT may show enhancing liver and nodal metastases, a stellate or spiculated mesenteric mass, scattered calcifications, bowel wall thickening, encasement of the vessels at the mesenteric root, and occasionally resultant ischemic bowel.

## ✓ Pearls & ✗ Pitfalls

✓ Carcinoid syndrome usually occurs in conjunction with multiple liver metastases and the release of serotonin, metabolites (flushing, cyanosis, sweating, watery diarrhea, cyanosis), and in severe cases right-sided congestive heart failure.

✓ Radiation enteritis can cause separation and tethering of small-bowel loops but typically affects all structures in the radiation field, not just a central focus of mesentery.

✗ Without carcinoid syndrome, small GI carcinoids are extremely difficult to distinguish from other submucosal masses.

✗ Percutaneous biopsy of liver metastasis may cause hypotensive crisis.

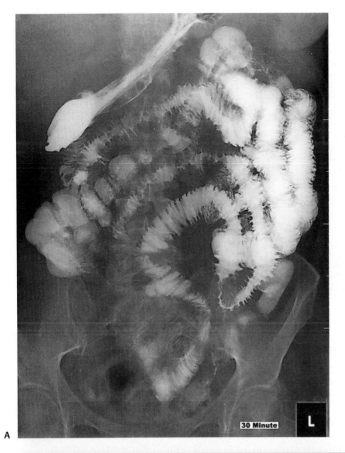

A

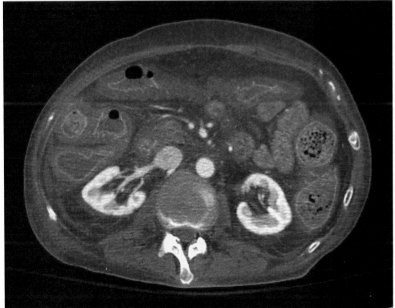

B

## Clinical Presentation

A 52-year-old woman presents with abdominal pain.

### ■ Imaging Findings

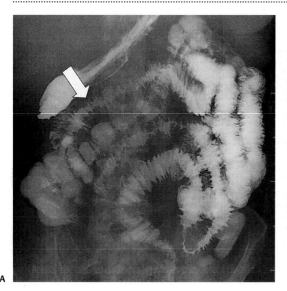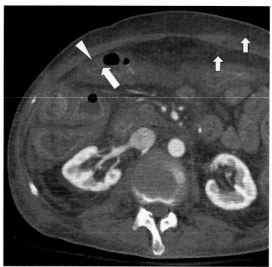

**(A)** Small-bowel follow-through shows diffuse, regularly thickened small-bowel folds (*arrow*). **(B)** Contrast-enhanced computed tomography (CT) in the arterial phase shows diffuse bowel wall thickening with a two-layer appearance: hyperdense mucosa (*arrow*) surrounded by a hypodense (water-density) submucosa (*arrowhead*). *Small arrows* indicate edematous fat.

### ■ Differential Diagnosis

- **Diffuse bowel wall edema:** This is the first diagnostic choice. Edematous mesenteric and subcutaneous fat can be caused by cirrhosis, renal failure, heart failure, or hypoproteinemia. This patient has abetalipoproteinemia.
- *Ischemic bowel:* This can present with these CT and barium findings, particularly with the "water halo" sign seen in this case. Thrombosis of the proximal superior mesenteric artery can also be present with this extensive distribution.
- *Venous congestion:* This is a third option that can cause edematous infiltration of the small and large bowel. Consider acute obstruction of mesenteric venous outflow from superior mesenteric, portal, or hepatic vein thrombosis.
- *Infectious enteritis (nonspecific):* This is less likely but can present with this pattern.

### ■ Essential Facts

- This case reviews the differential diagnosis for diffuse, regular thickening of small-bowel folds and the colon wall, as well as the CT pattern of the water halo sign. Although this differential is broad, the principal considerations are listed.

- Barium study findings:
  - Diffuse, regularly thickened small-bowel folds (> 3 mm) without malabsorption may be caused by arterial ischemia; mesenteric venous congestion/obstruction; hepatic, renal, or cardiac failure; infection; or acute radiation injury.
  - Hemorrhage can cause this pattern on barium studies. Consider hemophilia, Henoch-Schönlein purpura, or anticoagulation.
- CT findings:
  - The water halo sign is caused by a hypodense, water-density submucosa and a hyperdense mucosa (causing the two-layer pattern in this case), ± a hyperdense muscularis propria (all three layers, also called target sign).
  - The differential diagnosis for this pattern is broad and includes causes of acute bowel injury and edema.

### ✓ Pearls & ✗ Pitfalls

- ✓ The water halo or target sign is usually benign.
- ✓ For more focal presentations of regularly thickened small-bowel folds or the water halo sign, consider acute, focal inflammatory processes, such as infection or inflammatory bowel disease, acute bowel ischemia, and acute radiation enteritis.

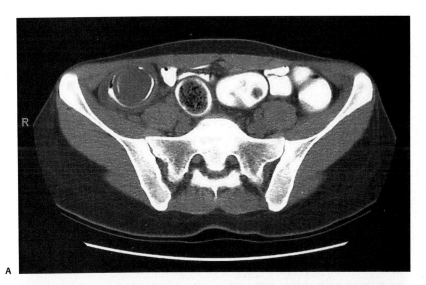

A

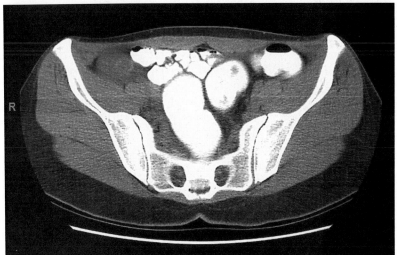

B

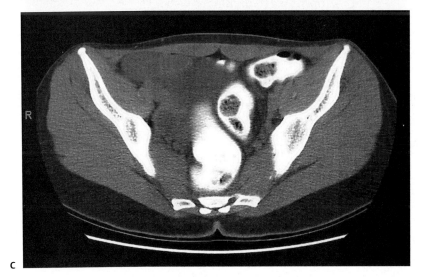

C

## ■ Clinical Presentation

A 26-year-old woman presents with fever and abdominal pain.

### ■ Imaging Findings

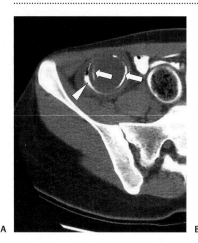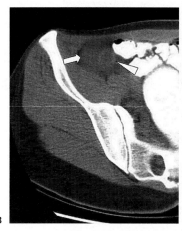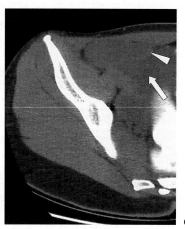

**(A)** Infused pelvic computed tomography (CT) with oral contrast shows a round, low-density structure with curvilinear rim calcifications (*arrows*) within the cecum, surrounded by barium (*arrowhead*). **(B)** Adjacent caudal image shows this structure (*arrow*) to abut a lower round structure (*arrowhead*) with a thick, enhancing wall and central low density. **(C)** More caudal image shows this second structure to be tubular (*arrowhead*) and surrounded by fluid (*arrow*).

### ■ Differential Diagnosis

• ***Appendiceal mucocele, intussusception, and appendicitis:*** This is the best explanation for this constellation of findings. The tubular structure is the dilated appendix with periappendiceal fluid, and the rounded structure is a mucocele of the base of the appendix that has prolapsed into the cecum, forming an intussusceptum.
•*Primary adenocarcinoma of the appendix or colon:* This may occasionally be cystic or cause cystic dilatation of the appendix, but rim calcifications are not characteristic, and this option is mentioned only for discussion.

### ■ Essential Facts

• *Appendiceal mucocele* is a basket term for any cystic mass of the appendix containing mucin. Appendiceal mucoceles are evident in 0.3% of resected appendix specimens.
• Mucoceles without complications typically appear on CT as round, fluid-density structures in the right lower quadrant, occasionally with rim calcifications. Associated inflammation of the appendix is seen in a minority of patients.
• Complications of mucoceles include intussusception, appendicitis (illustrated by this case), and rupture into the peritoneum.
• Subtypes are histopathologic:
  • Mucosal hyperplasia is often present in simple mucoceles, which may be caused by appendiceal obstruction from inflammation, lymphoid hyperplasia, or food.
  • Mucinous cystadenoma is the most common subtype, occurring in > 60% of cases.
  • Mucinous cystadenocarcinoma may be identical to benign mucoceles. Features suggesting malignancy are not always present and include enhancing nodules and invasion of adjacent structures.

• Pseudomyxoma peritonei (PP) can result from rupture of benign or malignant subtypes:
  • PP caused by cystadenoma carries an excellent long-term prognosis, but recurrence and bowel obstruction may develop after surgical evacuation.
  • PP caused by cystadenocarcinoma carries a 5-year survival rate of 25%.

### ■ Other Imaging Findings

• Ultrasound of benign mucoceles may show shadowing from rim calcifications and an anechoic center with increased through-transmission.
• Nodules or local invasion suggest but do not confirm malignancy.

### ✓ Pearls & ✗ Pitfalls

✓ PP can also be caused by ovarian mucinous cystadenocarcinoma (most commonly) and, rarely, by adenocarcinoma of the stomach, colon, and mucinous tumors of the pancreas.
✓ Carcinoid of the appendix is more common than mucocele and may cause obstruction and a cystic mass. Rim calcifications such as those seen in this case are not a characteristic feature.
✗ Surgical resection of mucoceles requires careful handling to avoid rupture and seeding of the peritoneum. Catheter drainage should be avoided!

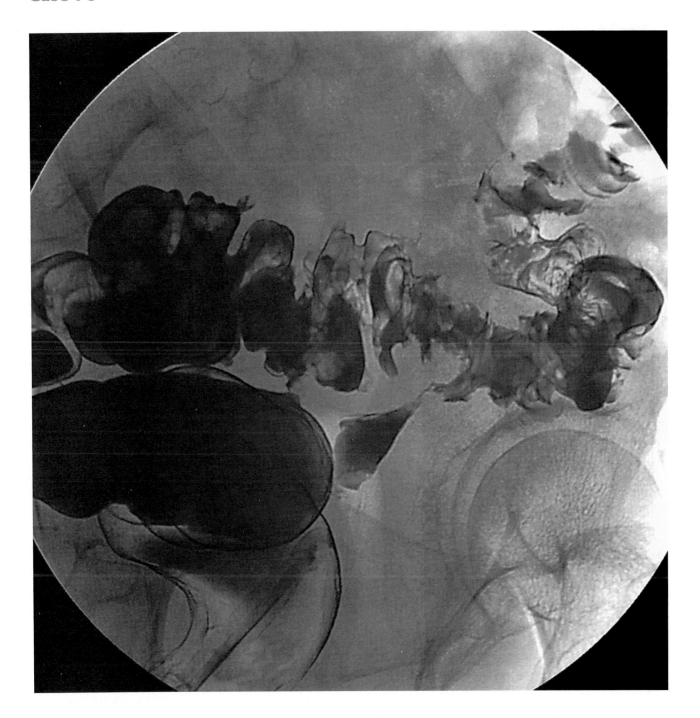

## Clinical Presentation

A 68-year-old woman presents with a past history of ovarian carcinoma.

### ■ Imaging Findings

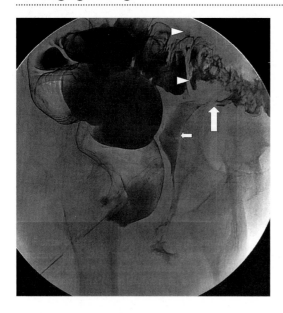

Dynamic proctography shows a single fistulous tract from the sigmoid colon to the vagina. Delayed image shows the fistula (*large arrow*), contrast in the vagina (*small arrow*), and leakage of contrast to the perineum. The sigmoid colon is circumferentially narrowed, and several diverticula are present (*arrowheads*).

### ■ Differential Diagnosis

- ***Diverticulitis causing colovaginal fistula:*** Sigmoid diverticula, diverticular disease (with circumferential luminal narrowing), and the proximity of the fistula to the abnormal segment of sigmoid colon place diverticulitis at the top of the list for diagnosis.
- *Malignancy:* This is a possible second; recurrence of the patient's ovarian cancer, new colon cancer, and other invasive pelvic neoplasms may cause fistulae.
- *Surgery:* Fistulae can be a complication of surgery; treatment for prior malignancy raises this possibility.
- *Radiation therapy:* The history of gynecologic malignancy raises this possibility, although radiation enteritis may have other findings not present: bowel wall effacement, rigidity, thickening, and tethering.

### ■ Essential Facts

- Diverticulosis describes focal outpouchings of colonic mucosa and submucosa through the muscularis mucosae at points of mesenteric vessel supply. These can occur throughout the colon but involve the sigmoid in > 95% of patients.
- Diverticulitis is focal infection due to perforation, which develops in 20% (most commonly sigmoid).
- Pericolic abscess occurs in one-third of cases of diverticulitis and fistula formation in < 10%.
- Causes of fistulae of the pelvis and abdomen:
  - Colovaginal: diverticulitis, malignancy, Crohn disease
  - Colovesical: diverticulitis, Crohn disease, trauma
  - Vesicovaginal: surgery (e.g., hysterectomy), malignancy (e.g., cervical), radiation
  - Vesicoenteric: Crohn disease, malignancy, trauma
- Clinical presentation of colovaginal fistula is usually foul-smelling vaginal discharge.

### ■ Other Imaging Findings

- Computed tomography (CT):
  - Best for suspected diverticulitis; look for diverticula, bowel wall thickening, pericolic fat stranding, or abscess
  - May demonstrate fistulae from bowel to enteric, gynecologic, or genitourinary structures. Rectal or oral contrast administration should be carefully timed to allow demonstration of the fistula itself or delayed leakage into the secondary structure.
- Cystography:
  - Cystography misses more than half of fistulae involving the bladder.
  - If cystography fails to show fistula, the indirect finding of gas in the bladder raises suspicion.

### ✓ Pearls & ✗ Pitfalls

- ✓ Fistulae may result from infectious, inflammatory, iatrogenic, and neoplastic processes. In addition to the common causes previously listed, consider appendicitis, abdominal abscesses, tuberculosis, and Crohn disease.
- ✓ Differential diagnosis should be rank-ordered based on the history, location, and imaging findings.
- ✗ Pelvic and abdominal fistulae may be missed in 50% of patients despite appropriate imaging via barium studies, cystography, and CT.
- ✗ Fistulae may be small, intermittent, or unidirectional, necessitating more than one study for visualization.

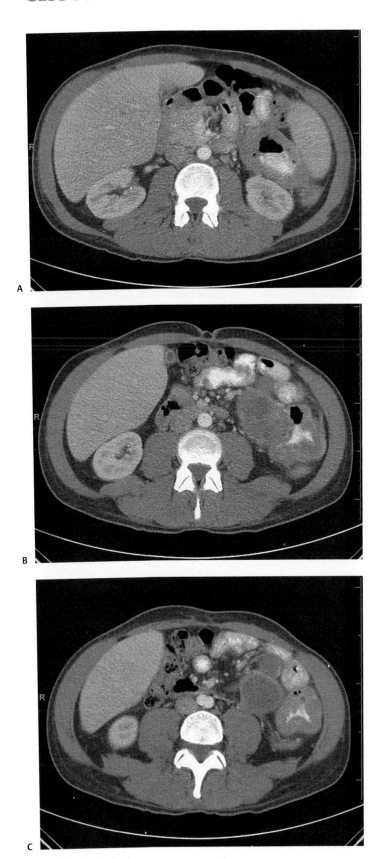

A

B

C

## ■ Clinical Presentation

A 39-year-old man presents with gastrointestinal bleeding.

## ■ Imaging Findings

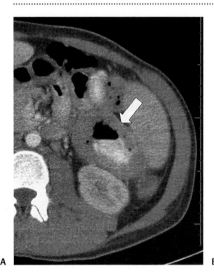
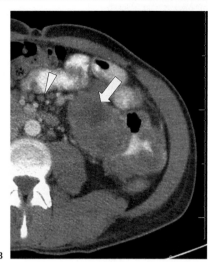
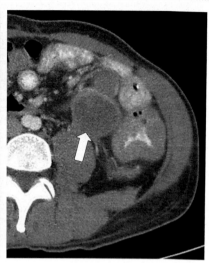

A                                   B                                   C

**(A)** Contrast-enhanced computed tomography shows marked, circumferential mural thickening (*arrow*) of the proximal jejunum and no enlarged lymph nodes. **(B)** More caudal image shows a large exophytic mass with central low-density areas of necrosis or cavitation (*arrow*). Minimal lymphadenopathy is noted (*arrowhead*). **(C)** More caudal image shows two lobulated components of the mass with an enhancing rim and central low density (*arrow*).

## ■ Differential Diagnosis

- **Melanoma:** This top diagnostic choice causes cavitary lesions of the small bowel, and metastatic disease is the most common small-bowel neoplasm.
- *Leiomyosarcoma:* This is the second option and can affect the small bowel with a large, exophytic, ulcerating mass in its exoenteric form.
- *Lymphoma:* A distant third, lymphoma causes marked small-bowel wall thickening in the infiltrative form and luminal dilatation, as seen in this case. This entity can also be polypoid and/or ulcerating; both features are present in this case. However, the absence of local or remote lymphadenopathy is less characteristic of lymphoma.
- *Primary adenocarcinoma of the small bowel:* This is uncommon and more often presents with stricture from focal, irregularly marginated, annular wall thickening, occasionally with nodal metastases. Cavitation and large exophytic masses are possible, but unlikely.

## ■ Essential Facts

- The key to this case is rank-ordering neoplasms of the small bowel that cause large exophytic masses and cavitation or central necrosis.
- Malignant melanoma affects the small bowel in < 10% of metastatic cases.
- More common sites of metastasis are the liver, lungs, adrenal glands, and kidneys. Necrosis, cavitation, and ulceration are common in any location.
- Clinical presentation of gastrointestinal (GI) involvement is often GI bleeding due to ulceration and hypervascularity.

- Imaging findings of GI melanoma:
  - Classically: multiple submucosal polyps with central ulceration
  - Alternatively: large, exophytic mass that is cavitary, necrotic, or ulcerated
  - Masses and associated lymphadenopathy tend to have the common feature of enhancing tissue surrounding low-density cavitation or necrosis.

## ■ Other Imaging Findings

- Barium studies may show multiple polyps with central barium collections (bull's-eye lesions).

## ✓ Pearls & ✗ Pitfalls

- ✓ Leiomyosarcoma of the small bowel affects the ileum > jejunum > duodenum.
  - Most are large, exophytic, and centrally necrotic on presentation.
  - Diffuse mural infiltration and intraluminal polyp formation are much less common.
- ✓ Lymphoma of the small bowel also affects the ileum > jejunum > duodenum.
  - Diffuse mural infiltration is more common than exophytic masses or intraluminal polyps.
  - A distinguishing feature is small-bowel aneurysmal dilatation.
  - Bulky mesenteric nodes with minimal or no enhancement may become a confluent mass.

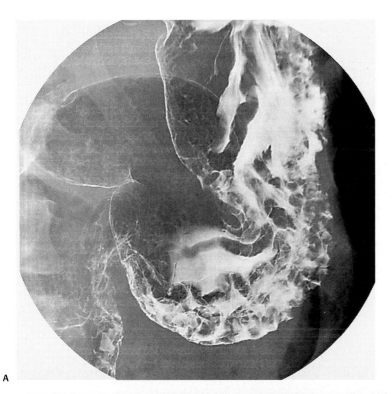

A

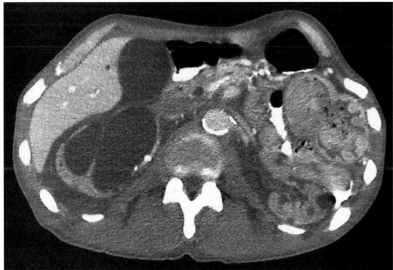

B

## Clinical Presentation

A 63-year-old man with end-stage renal disease presents with midepigastric pain.

### Imaging Findings

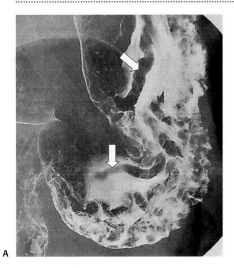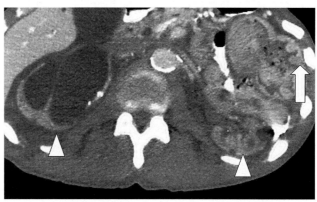

**(A)** Upper gastrointestinal barium study shows diffusely thickened rugal folds (*arrows*) despite adequate distension. **(B)** Contrast-enhanced computed tomography (CT) shows thickened rugal folds (*arrow*) and atrophic kidneys (*arrowheads*) with cysts.

### Differential Diagnosis

- ***Chronic gastritis from renal failure:*** This is at the top of the list because of the history of renal failure and diffuse, uniform gastric fold thickening.
- *Gastritis* (Helicobacter pylori*)*: This is second as this entity is the most common cause of rugal fold thickening.
- *Ménétrier disease:* Expect hypersecretion and possible antral sparing, both present in this case.
- *Zollinger-Ellison syndrome:* Expect hypersecretion, small-bowel involvement, and evidence of gastrinoma.

### Essential Facts

- Patients with chronic renal failure who are on dialysis may have hypergastrinemia producing hyperchlorhydria and resulting in gastritis, peptic ulcer disease, and/or gastrointestinal bleeding.
- Gastritis (*H. pylori*) is the most common cause of gastric fold thickening. It is typically mild to moderate and regular. It may be focal (typically antral) or diffuse.
- Zollinger-Ellison syndrome may present with an enhancing pancreatic mass (gastrinoma), fold thickening involving the stomach, proximal small-bowel ulcers, and hypersecretion.
- Ménétrier disease may present with fold thickening—typically massive and lobulated—sparing the antrum in 50%. Loss of parietal and chief cells results in hypochlorhydria and hypersecretion.
- Malignancy such as lymphoma or adenocarcinoma is variable in appearance but may present with disorganized fold thickening, nodularity due to submucosal spread, and poor distensibility.
- Eosinophilic gastritis may present with diffuse fold thickening in the stomach and small bowel associated with allergy.

- Pancreatic pathology such as pancreatitis, malignancy, abscess, or pseudocyst may cause adjacent fold thickening that is typically focal.
- Portal hypertensive gastropathy may have finely nodular fold thickening.

### Other Imaging Findings

- Barium studies: details that may hone the differential diagnosis of rugal fold thickening include the presence of hypersecretion, distensibility, focal versus diffuse thickening, regular versus disorganized thickening, and the degree and quality of thickening (including mild, moderate, or severe and polypoid or lobulated).
- CT may hone the differential diagnosis by the presence of enhancing masses (pancreas or liver) to suggest gastrinoma and the presence of lymphadenopathy to suggest lymphoma or adenocarcinoma.

### ✓ Pearls & ✗ Pitfalls

- ✓ Mucosal or submucosal infiltration can cause rugal fold thickening, and different conditions may be indistinguishable by barium study and CT.
- ✓ Differential diagnosis for rugal thickening includes benign conditions such as gastritis, pancreatitis, eosinophilic gastritis, Ménétrier disease, Zollinger-Ellison syndrome, and portal hypertensive gastropathy, as well as malignancies such as lymphoma, adenocarcinoma, and pancreatic carcinoma.
- ✓ Endoscopic biopsy may be required for diagnosis.
- ✗ Gastric varices may mimic fold thickening but are typically smooth, tortuous, often fundal (extending into the esophagus), and often associated with liver failure.

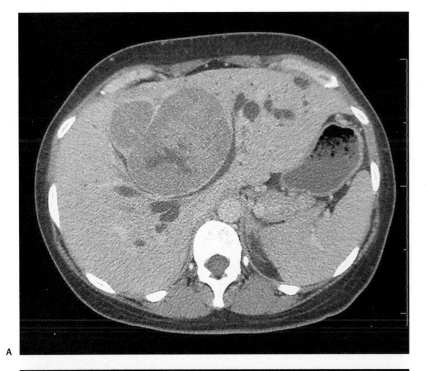

A

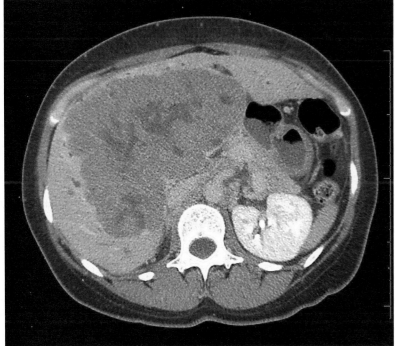

B

## ■ Clinical Presentation

A 35-year-old woman presents with right upper quadrant pain. Her α-fetoprotein level is normal.

## ■ Imaging Findings

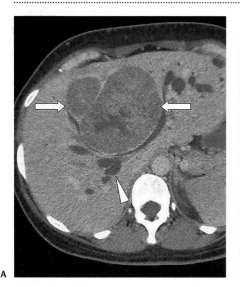
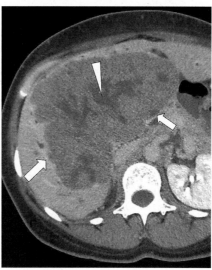

**(A)** Infused abdominal computed tomography (CT) shows a well-circumscribed, heterogeneous hepatic mass (*arrows*) that is hypodense to liver parenchyma and obstructs the intrahepatic bile ducts (*arrowhead*). **(B)** More caudal image shows the mass to be quite large, with a lobulated contour (*large arrow*), a dense capsule (*small arrow*), and a hypodense, radiating central region (*arrowhead*).

## ■ Differential Diagnosis

- **Fibrolamellar carcinoma (FLC):** This top choice is suggested by a large, encapsulated mass with a hypodense central scar on delayed imaging and a lobulated contour in a young patient. The α-fetoprotein level is typically normal, as in this case.
- *Hepatic adenoma:* A less likely conclusion in this case, although a history of oral contraceptives might raise this entity to the top of the list. These lesions can be quite large and present with an enhancing capsule and a central scar due to necrosis. Look for draped peripheral vessels.
- *Focal nodular hyperplasia (FNH):* FNH is worthy of consideration for a hepatic mass with a central scar in a young adult. The central scar tends to enhance more brightly than the periphery of the lesion on delayed imaging.

## ■ Essential Facts

- FLC is a malignant tumor of the hepatocytes with a propensity to develop central lamellar fibrosis that sometimes results in the appearance of a central scar.
- Unlike standard hepatocellular carcinoma (HCC), FLC occurs in a younger age group (5–35 years), typically without associated cirrhosis.
- Imaging findings typically include lobulated margins (as in this case), a dense capsule, and a central scar that remains hypodense on all phases of CT. Calcifications are common.
- CT usually shows heterogeneous enhancement of FLC in the arterial phase and earlier washout of contrast compared with liver parenchyma, similar to HCC.

## ■ Other Imaging Findings

- Magnetic resonance imaging (MRI) of FLC shows the mass to have decreased signal on T1 and increased signal on T2. The scar shows decreased signal on T1, T2, and enhanced images.
- Sulfur colloid uptake is one way to distinguish FLC (negative) from FNH (may be positive).

## ✓ Pearls & ✗ Pitfalls

- ✓ Cholangiocarcinoma may present as a large, solitary intrahepatic mass, but lacking the dense capsule seen in this case. Look for irregular margins, hepatic capsular retraction, and delayed washout of contrast in these lesions.
- ✓ Unlike FLC, hepatic adenoma is more homogeneous (unless hemorrhage has occurred), is related to oral contraceptive and steroid use, typically has draped peripheral vessels, and is usually more smoothly marginated.
- ✓ Unlike FLC, FNH does not calcify and has delayed enhancement on MRI and CT in the central scar due to hypervascularity.
- ✗ FLC, hepatic adenoma, and FNH have overlapping clinical and imaging features, including presentation in young adults without cirrhosis and the presence of a central scar.
- ✗ Evaluation of enhancement patterns, contour, and vascularity may help distinguish these entities.

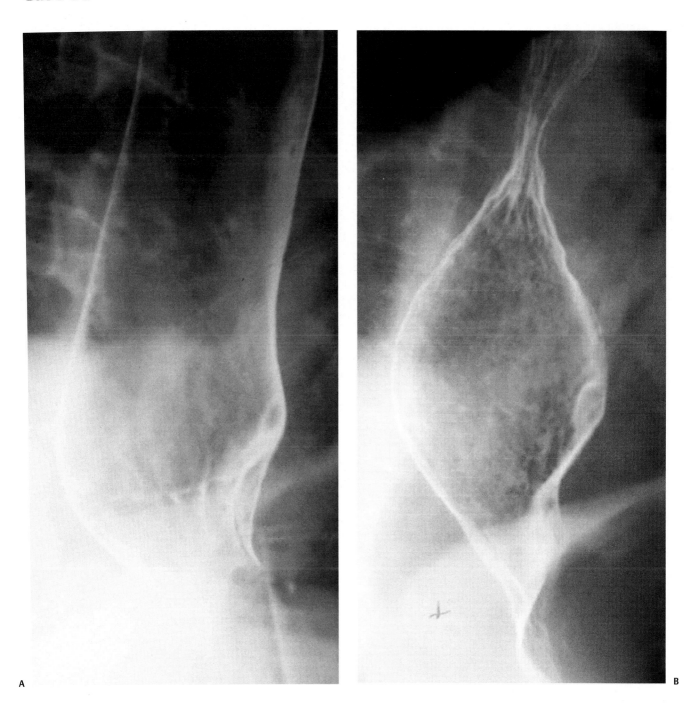

A

B

## Clinical Presentation

A 35-year-old man presents to the gastroenterology clinic with chronic, mild midepigastric pain.

## ■ Imaging Findings

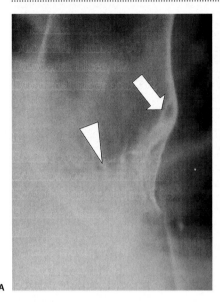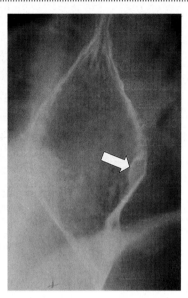

**(A)** Double-contrast esophagogram shows a prominent squamocolumnar mucosal junction (Z line; *arrowhead*) and a small submucosal mass (*arrow*) at this level. **(B)** The mass (*arrow*) is well circumscribed and makes obtuse angles with the esophageal wall, identifying it as submucosal.

## ■ Differential Diagnosis

- *Leiomyoma:* This is the most likely diagnosis for a smoothly marginated, submucosal (intramural) esophageal mass, based purely on statistical probability. The imaging findings are nonspecific.
- *Neural tumor:* Schwannoma, neurofibroma, or granular cell tumor may be submucosal. Neurofibromas typically occur in patients with von Recklinghausen disease.
- *Other benign tumors of the esophagus:* These may be submucosal, including lipoma, fibroma, hamartoma, and hemangioma. The exact incidence of these lesions in the esophagus is unclear, but they are typically included in the differential diagnosis of a submucosal mass.

## ■ Essential Facts

- This case reviews the differential diagnosis for a small submucosal mass of the esophagus and demonstrates the squamocolumnar mucosal junction (Z line).
- Leiomyoma is a slow-growing, benign spindle cell tumor rich in smooth-muscle cells.
- Most tumors of the esophagus are malignant (99%). Most benign tumors are leiomyomas (50–67%).
- Clinical presentation: leiomyomas of the esophagus are usually asymptomatic, incidental findings, but larger lesions may present with dysphagia; ulcerated lesions may present with pain and upper gastrointestinal bleeding.
- Imaging findings typical of a leiomyoma:
  - Smooth margination indicating intact overlying mucosa (ulceration possible but uncommon)

- Usually located in the middle to lower esophagus as this region contains predominantly smooth rather than striated muscle
- May be very large or multiple
- Follow-up may include long-range serial imaging studies as a very low risk for malignant degeneration to leiomyosarcoma does exist.
- Treatment is most commonly open surgical resection. Endoscopic resection has been described.

## ■ Other Imaging Findings

- Computed tomography (CT) of esophageal leiomyomas shows diffuse enhancement and occasional calcifications. Other esophageal tumors do not calcify.

## ✓ Pearls & ✗ Pitfalls

- ✓ Alport syndrome is a genetic syndrome consisting predominantly of deafness, glomerulonephritis, and renal failure. Patients are predisposed to diffuse leiomyomatosis of the esophagus.
- ✓ Duplication cysts are congenital cystic lesions appearing as a submucosal mass on barium studies and a homogeneous low-density mass on CT. They are typically larger at presentation than the lesion shown in this case.
- ✗ Early esophageal cancer originates in the epithelium but may appear as a small, well-defined mass in some cases. Either adenocarcinoma or squamous cell carcinoma can originate from the squamocolumnar junction.

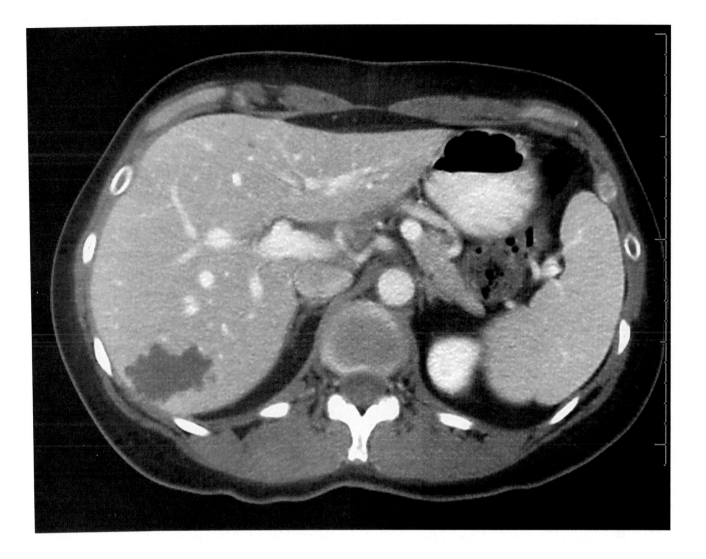

## Clinical Presentation

A 45-year-old woman presents with right upper quadrant pain without fever or leukocytosis.

## Imaging Findings

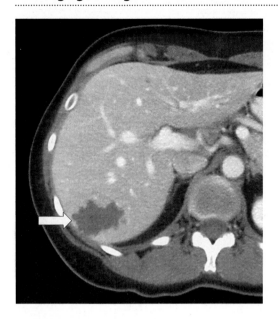

Contrast-enhanced computed tomography (CT) shows a well-circumscribed, multiloculated cystic lesion (*arrow*) in the right lobe of the liver. No enhancing nodular components are visible. Scattered, smaller low-density foci are seen in the liver, most likely cysts.

## Differential Diagnosis

- **Biliary cystadenoma:** This is the strongest contender as the diagnosis for a multiloculated, smoothly marginated cystic lesion in the liver without clinical signs of infection.
- *Hepatic cyst:* This can have a similar appearance in a minority of cases. This patient has other low-density lesions suspicious for simple cysts.
- *Echinococcal cyst:* This often results from infection by *Echinococcus granulosus* or *Echinococcus multilocularis* and may present as a multiloculated cystic lesion with a lobulated contour caused by budding daughter cysts at the periphery of the lesion.
- *Abscess (pyogenic):* This may have the CT appearance of the "cluster" sign, evidenced by a multiloculated cluster of small fluid collections; however, the clinical presentation is not suggestive. This entity would be suggested by round, septated collections with debris/gas, an enhancing wall, and a surrounding rim of edema.

## Essential Facts

- Biliary cystadenoma is a benign tumor of bile duct origin with mucin-containing cysts that most commonly presents in middle age. Malignant degeneration to biliary cystadenocarcinoma is possible.
- Clinical presentation is usually pain, abdominal distension, or an incidental discovery in an asymptomatic individual, as in this case. Very large lesions can compress adjacent abdominal structures.
- Imaging findings are variable, but generally:
  - Uniloculated or multiloculated, smoothly marginated cystic mass that can be quite large
  - Variable fluid characteristics depending on the levels of blood, bile, or mucin

- Nodularity or papillary projections are suggestive, but not indicative, of degeneration to biliary cystadenocarcinoma.
- Treatment for biliary cystadenoma is surgical resection because of the malignant potential and symptoms related to the expansile nature of these lesions. Partial resection may lead to recurrence, even in benign cases.

## Other Imaging Findings

- Magnetic resonance imaging of:
  - Biliary cystadenoma shows homogeneous low signal intensity (SI) on T1 and high SI on T2.
  - Echinococcal cysts may show the "water lily" sign of curvilinear internal membranes.

## ✓ Pearls & ✗ Pitfalls

- ✓ Ovarian stroma may be present in cystadenocarcinoma in women, a subtype that carries a better prognosis.
- ✓ Echinococcal cysts (tapeworm larvae) may be uniloculated with rim calcification but more often present as a multiloculated, complex lesion that resembles a cystic neoplasm. They expand and propagate with internal daughter cysts and budding cysts.
- ✓ Mesenchymal hamartoma can be indistinguishable from biliary cystadenoma on imaging studies but typically presents in childhood.
- ✗ Slow growth can occur with both biliary cystadenoma and hepatic cysts, making them indistinguishable on serial imaging studies in many cases.
- ✗ Cystic hepatocellular carcinoma or hepatic metastases can mimic biliary cystadenoma or cystadenocarcinoma.

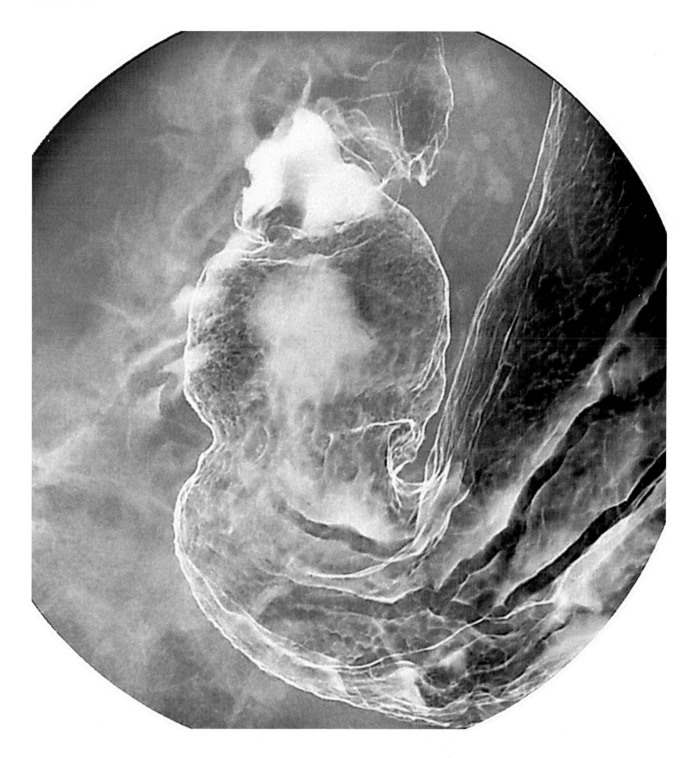

## ■ Clinical Presentation

A 35-year-old woman presents with midepigastric pain.

■ **Imaging Findings**

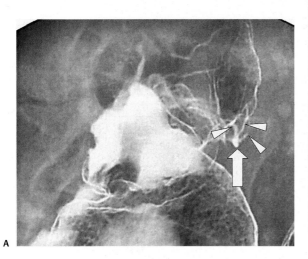
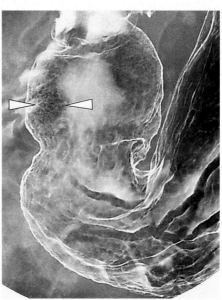

A                                                                            B

**(A)** Double-contrast barium study of the duodenal bulb shows a pit of barium extending beyond the confines of the lumen (*arrow*). Several radiating folds (*arrowheads*) filled with barium extend into this pit, and there is mild deformity of the bulb, particularly near the pit. **(B)** The areae gastricae (*arrowheads*) are diffusely prominent throughout the gastric lumen.

■ **Differential Diagnosis**

• ***Duodenal ulcer scar caused by prior peptic ulcer disease:*** This is the most likely diagnosis for a pit of barium in the duodenal bulb with associated radiating folds and mild retraction of the adjacent wall.
• *Duodenal ulcer:* The less likely choice, as one would expect an adjacent mound of edematous tissue and more edematous, thickened radiating folds.

■ **Essential Facts**

• Duodenal ulcers are more common in men and:
  • Are not premalignant.
  • Are usually small (< 1 cm) and singular, and occur in patients with deformity of the bulb due to chronic peptic ulcer disease.
  • Are giant (> 2 cm) in a minority of cases (increased risk for bleeding and marked scarring).
  • Commonly occur on the anterior wall of the bulb, making prone views critical for demonstrating pooling in the crater and radiating folds. Supine double-contrast views may show a ring shadow of barium around the ulcer crater, as seen in gastric ulcers.
• Duodenal ulcers and enlarged areae gastricae have a strong association with infection by *Helicobacter pylori*, which is treatable with antibiotics.

✓ **Pearls & ✗ Pitfalls**

✓ Zollinger-Ellison syndrome (ZES) is caused by hypersecretion of gastric acid due to a gastrinoma. ZES may cause ulcers in both the gastric antrum and duodenum, usually in the bulb (95%).
✓ Postbulbar ulcers occur almost exclusively with ZES syndrome but still represent only 5% of duodenal ulcers associated with ZES.
✗ Scarring may mimic an active ulcer, as in this case. The classic example of scarring from healed peptic ulcer disease is the so-called cloverleaf deformity.
✗ Active ulcers may mimic scarring, particular giant ulcers that may be mistaken for gross bulb deformity.

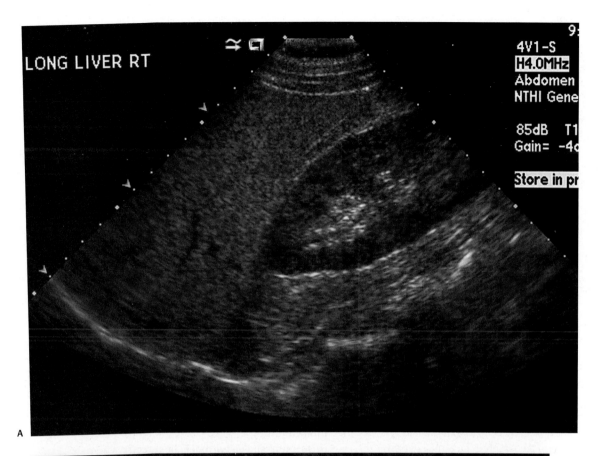

A

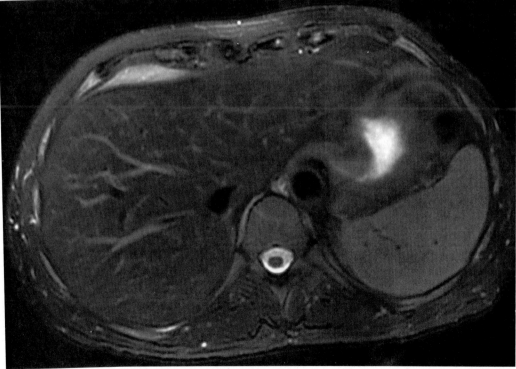

B

■ **Clinical Presentation**

A 54-year-old man presents for further work-up of an incidental finding on abdominal ultrasound.

## ■ Imaging Findings

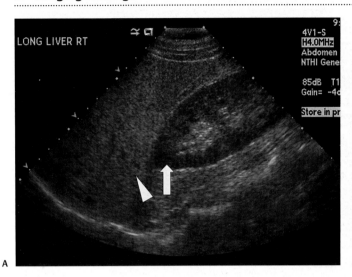
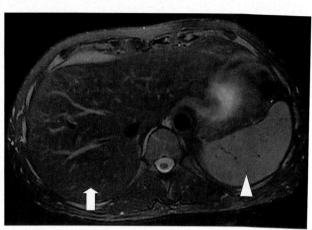

**(A)** Ultrasound shows diffuse, coarse echogenicity of the liver parenchyma (*arrowhead*) compared with the normal-appearing kidney parenchyma (*arrow*).
**(B)** T2-weighted magnetic resonance imaging (MRI) shows a homogeneously hypointense liver (*arrow*) compared with the normal-appearing spleen (*arrowhead*).

### ■ Differential Diagnosis

- **Hemochromatosis (primary):** The top diagnosis, it classically causes markedly decreased signal intensity (SI) on T2-weighted MRI and a coarsely echogenic liver on ultrasound due to hepatic fibrosis.
- *Fatty infiltration of the liver:* This may show decreased signal on T2 (to a lesser degree) and markedly decreased signal on T2 fat saturation images. The liver is also echogenic.

### ■ Essential Facts

- Hemochromatosis may be primary or secondary and results in increased iron deposition in tissues.
- Primary:
  - An autosomal-recessive intestinal disorder resulting in increased iron absorption and iron deposition predominantly within the hepatocytes rather than the Kupffer cells
  - Causes fibrosis, cirrhosis, and an increased risk for hepatocellular carcinoma (HCC)
  - Associated features include hyperpigmentation, diabetes, hepatomegaly, osteoarthritis, and cardiomyopathy.
  - Ultrasound shows coarse echogenicity.
  - MRI shows markedly decreased T2 gradient-echo SI predominantly in the liver and *pancreas* (SI < muscle), reflecting preferential organ involvement.
- Secondary:
  - Acquired condition in which iron deposits primarily in the Kupffer cells with no associated hepatic damage

- Rarely clinically significant
- Causes include multiple blood transfusions, sickle cell anemia, and Bantu siderosis, which is excessive dietary intake of iron.
- Ultrasound shows normal echogenicity.
- MRI features are similar to those of primary hemochromatosis except that the decreased SI occurs predominantly in the liver and *spleen* (SI < muscle), reflecting preferential organ involvement.

### ■ Other Imaging Findings

- Fatty infiltration is sometimes distinguishable by characteristic fat-sparing regions (near gallbladder or in caudate) and only mild to moderate decrease in T2 SI.
- Computed tomography of hemochromatosis shows nonspecific diffuse hyperattenuation in the liver.

### ✓ Pearls & ✗ Pitfalls

- ✓ Do not miss HCC on cross-sectional imaging in cases of primary hemochromatosis.
- ✓ Diffuse echogenic or hyperattenuating liver may be caused by a host of differential possibilities, including deposition of proteins or glycogen (storage diseases), iodine (amiodarone), copper (Wilson disease), and gold (treatment for rheumatoid arthritis).

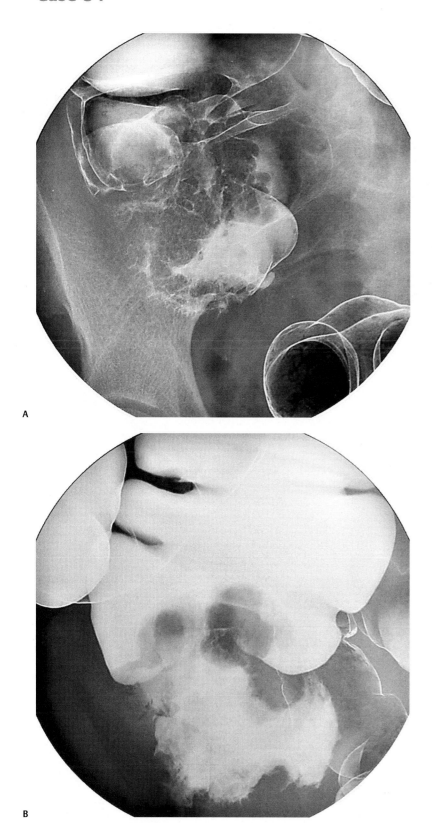

A

B

## Clinical Presentation

A 69-year-old woman presents with chronic, intermittent lower gastrointestinal bleeding.

## ■ Imaging Findings

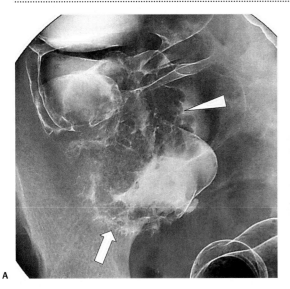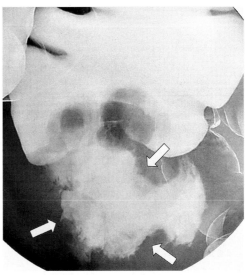

**(A)** Double-contrast barium study shows a multilobulated mass in the cecum with a smoothly marginated, nodular component (*arrowhead*) and a fronded, villous, soft-tissue proliferation (*arrow*) extending around the right lateral and inferior cecum. **(B)** Single-contrast study accentuates this villous component (*arrows*).

## ■ Differential Diagnosis

- **Villous adenoma:** This classic entity is associated with a carpet lesion. The associated lobulated mass may be a portion of the adenoma or colon carcinoma.
- *Invasive adenocarcinoma:* This second option spreads submucosally and extends intraluminally, causing the appearance of a carpet lesion.

## ■ Essential Facts

- The key to this case is having a good differential diagnosis for a carpet lesion of the colon at the ready.
- Carpet lesions are benign or malignant, nodular or fronded abnormalities that involve the superficial surface of any segment of the colonic lumen.
- Villous adenoma is the classic carpet lesion, but tubular and tubulovillous histologic types can also cause this appearance. The high potential for malignant degeneration of villous adenomas makes the detection and characterization of carpet lesions critical.

- Focal segmental nodularity from colitis or Crohn disease can present as a carpet lesion.
- Submucosal varices can present as clusters of nodules when seen en face.
- Endometriosis is focal and associated with crenulations that can appear carpetlike in tangential view and distorted, crinkled, or nodular en face.
- Polyposis caused by entities such as familial adenomatous polyposis is typically not confused with villous adenomas because of a known clinical history and imaging appearance.

## ✓ Pearls & ✗ Pitfalls

✓ Colonic urticaria is usually distinguishable from a carpet lesion by a characteristic polygonal mosaic of mucosal mounds separated by thin lines containing barium. This entity may result from marked colonic dilatation, allergy, herpes, Yersinia infection, Crohn disease, or ischemic bowel.

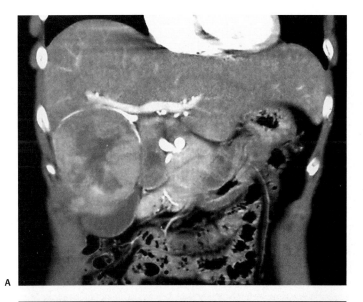

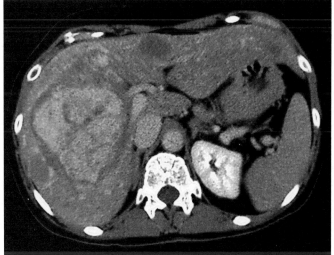

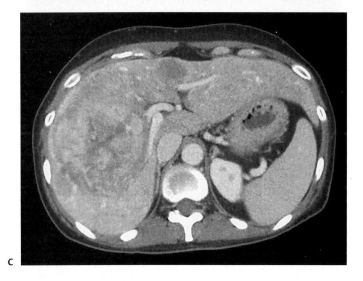

## ▣ Clinical Presentation

...........................................................................................................................................................................

A 50-year-old woman presents with abdominal pain and an enlarged liver on physical examination.

## Imaging Findings

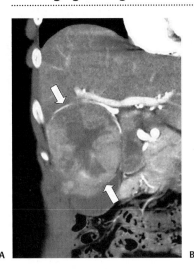
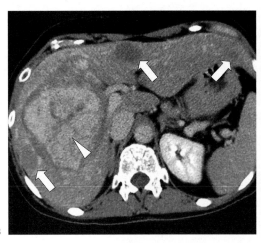
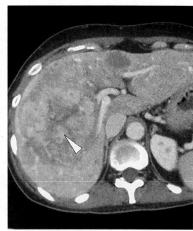

**(A)** Coronal, enhanced computed tomography (CT) image in the arterial phase shows a large, heterogeneous mass (*arrows*) in the right lobe of the liver. The peripheral portions of the mass enhance similarly to liver parenchyma, but the enhancement is variable, with peripheral hyperattenuating and central hypoattenuating regions. **(B)** Delayed imaging shows the mass to be hyperattenuating compared with normal liver, with delayed enhancement of the central regions (*arrowhead*). Additional hypoattenuating lesions are visible (*arrows*) and demonstrate peripherally draped vessels. **(C)** Portal venous-phase image shows delayed washout of contrast from the bulk of the mass, particularly the central regions (*arrowhead*).

## Differential Diagnosis

- **Hepatic adenoma (telangiectatic):** This diagnosis is most likely, given the finding of a large, relatively well-circumscribed, heterogeneously enhancing mass in the liver with peripherally draped vessels.
- *Hepatocellular carcinoma (HCC; in particular, fibrolamellar subtype):* HCC is the less likely choice because of the limited arterial-phase enhancement and the presence of vascular displacement rather than encasement or invasion.
- *Cholangiocarcinoma:* This may present with a large intrahepatic mass and delayed washout of contrast, but the imaging features are usually different (including vascular invasion, indistinct margins, earlier enhancement, and capsular retraction).
- *Hemangioma:* This is unlikely but is mentioned because of the delayed central enhancement and washout. The variable enhancement of large regions of the mass in the arterial phase makes this choice less likely.

## Essential Facts

- This case is an unusual presentation of hepatic adenoma that tests your ability to formulate a differential diagnosis in the face of imaging findings that are atypical for most hepatic neoplasms. In such a case, it is important to include a brief qualifying statement with each diagnostic possibility.
- Hepatic adenomas are benign neoplasms originating from hepatocytes that most typically occur in young adult women on oral contraceptives (OCs) or patients on other steroids.

- Imaging studies usually show a large (mean of 9 cm), solitary, heterogeneous mass reflecting regions of necrosis and hemorrhage. CT of adenomas usually shows early enhancement and washout, but this case shows both typical and atypical features of hepatic adenoma.
- Typical features include draped peripheral vessels, heterogeneous density, and large size.
- Atypical features include variable enhancement in the arterial phase, delayed enhancement, and washout of large central regions and multiple additional masses (see "Pearls & Pitfalls").
- Complications of adenomas include pain, bleeding, rupture, and malignant degeneration (to HCC).
- Treatment is surgical excision because of the risk for malignant degeneration.

## ✓ Pearls & ✗ Pitfalls

- ✓ Multiple hepatic adenomas may occur in women on OCs or with disorders of increased estrogen.
- ✓ Hepatocellular adenomatosis is multiple adenomas unrelated to estrogen levels and OCs; it may occur in both men and women.
- ✓ Telangiectatic adenomas have prominent vascular features that cause focal areas of delayed contrast enhancement and washout in a manner more similar to hemangioma than hepatic adenoma. This case is a telangiectatic adenoma.
- ✗ When imaging features are atypical, maintain a broad differential and recommend a confirmatory biopsy.

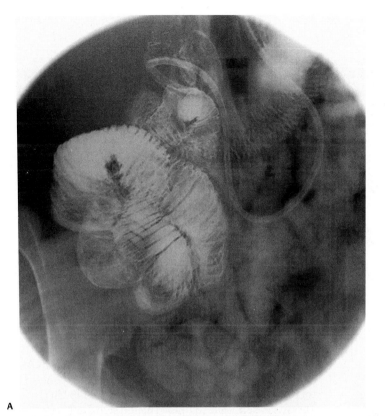

A

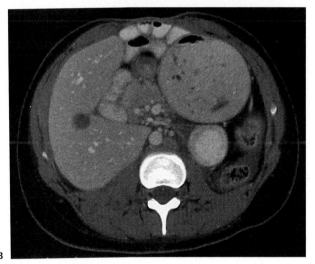

B

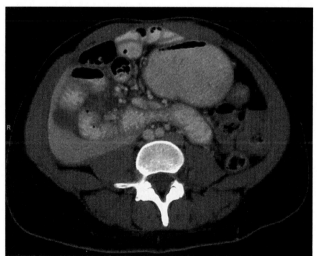

C

## ▪ Clinical Presentation

......................................................................................................................................................

An 18-year-old woman presents to the gastroenterology clinic with chronic, intermittent abdominal pain.

## ▓ Imaging Findings

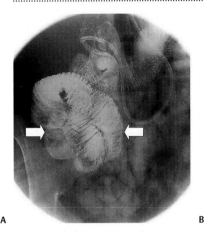
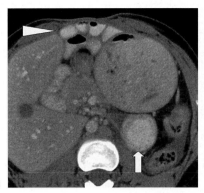
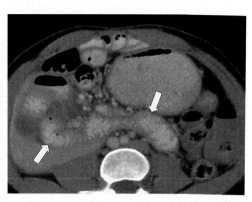

**(A)** Small-bowel series shows multiple jejunal loops (*arrows*) within the right hemiabdomen, indicating malrotation. **(B)** Contrast-enhanced computed tomography (CT) shows a dilated loop of small bowel in the left hemiabdomen with mural thickening (*arrow*) and multiple small-bowel loops in the anterior right hemiabdomen (*arrowhead*). **(C)** The thickened loop leads into an anomalous jejunal course (*arrows*), crossing the midline adjacent to the duodenum and behind the superior mesenteric artery (fossa of Waldeyer) and continuing as multiple loops in the right hemiabdomen.

## ▓ Differential Diagnosis

- ***Paraduodenal (right) hernia:*** Paraduodenal (right) hernia with resulting malrotation is the most likely choice of diagnosis, given the thickened small-bowel loop and the abnormally positioned small bowel.
- *Malrotation:* This is a possibility for the fluoroscopic study, but the CT findings and symptoms suggest herniation with ischemic changes.

## ▓ Essential Facts

- Internal hernias result from congenital, traumatic, or post-surgical herniation of bowel through a space completely contained within the peritoneal sac. They are much less common than external hernias.
- Presentation varies from asymptomatic to intermittent bowel obstruction to bowel ischemia from volvulus and/or strangulation.
- Types include paraduodenal, lesser sac, and much less commonly small-bowel mesentery, pericecal and sigmoid mesentery, and broad ligament of the pelvis.
- Paraduodenal:
  - Occurs through a rent between the mesentery and parietal peritoneum at the ligament of Treitz and is the most common type
  - Small bowel herniates into the left (most commonly) or right hemiabdomen and transverse mesocolon, displacing the transverse colon downward.
  - Right paraduodenal hernias (fossa of Waldeyer) occur with incomplete malrotation. The duodenal-jejunal junction is low and to the right of the midline, and multiple jejunal loops are in the right hemiabdomen.
  - Left paraduodenal hernias (fossa of Landzert) result in a mass of dilated small bowel in the left upper quadrant, lateral to the 4th portion of the duodenum.

- Lesser sac:
  - Occurs through the foramen of Winslow and is a surgical emergency due to impending strangulation of herniated small or large bowel, omentum, or gallbladder
  - Lesser sac hernias result in herniated structures posteromedially along the lesser curvature of the stomach, displacing the stomach and transverse colon downward and to the left.
- Pericecal hernias include ileocolic, retrocecal, ileocecal, and retroappendiceal types.
- Treatment of internal hernias is typically surgical reduction and closure of the internal rent.

## ▓ Other Imaging Findings

- CT of lesser sac hernias shows structures passing through the foramen of Winslow into the lesser sac, posterior to the stomach and caudate lobe and anterior to the pancreas, transverse colon, and mesocolon.
- CT of left paraduodenal hernias shows a confined mass of small-bowel loops to the left of the ligament of Treitz, between the lateral aspects of the stomach and pancreas.

## ✓ Pearls & ✗ Pitfalls

- ✓ As in this case, internal hernias may be associated with incomplete intestinal malrotation and contain variable amounts of bowel.
- ✓ Depending on the type of hernia, both large and small bowel may be involved.
- ✗ Internal hernias can be missed during imaging studies and at surgery if they are small and/or intermittent.
- ✗ If incarcerated, internal hernias may appear as multiple fluid-filled structures or air-fluid levels, mimicking abdominal abscesses. Do not miss pneumatosis indicating ischemic bowel!

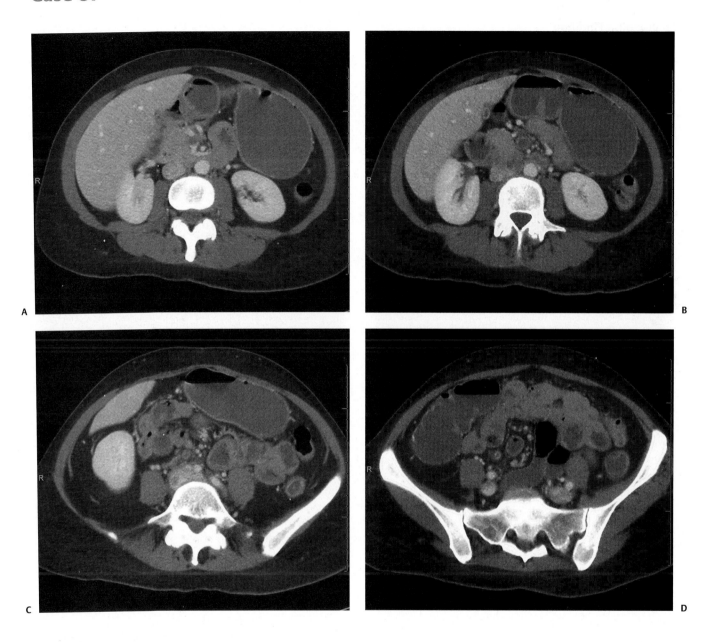

## Clinical Presentation

A 39-year-old woman presents with 1 week of increasing abdominal pain, fever, nausea, and vomiting.

### ■ Imaging Findings

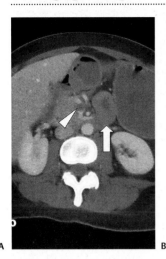
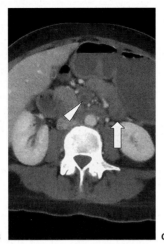
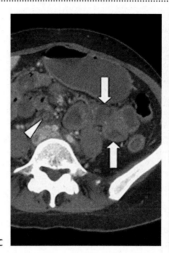
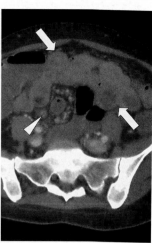

**(A)** Contrast-enhanced computed tomography (CT) shows thrombus (*arrowhead*) at the confluence of the splenic and portal veins. The duodenal wall is markedly thickened (*arrow*) with a diffusely hyperdense pattern (also called the white attenuation pattern). **(B)** More caudal image shows thrombus (*arrowhead*) filling the superior mesenteric vein (SMV). Small-bowel (SB) wall thickening (*arrow*) is seen. **(C)** More caudal image shows more distal thrombus (*arrowhead*) in the SMV and distended jejunal loops (*arrows*) with marked mural thickening demonstrating the uniform white attenuation pattern. **(D)** Thrombus extends into peripheral branches (*arrowhead*), and thickened SB appears coalesced and masslike (*arrows*).

### ■ Differential Diagnosis

- **SMV thrombosis:** This is evidenced by the filling defect coursing throughout the SMV and its branches and the slow onset of symptoms. SMV thrombosis can be primary or secondary.
  - *Secondary to an underlying condition:* This is to be considered in tandem with the first diagnosis. Although SB thickening is a feature of SMV thrombosis, the appearance in this case is somewhat atypical, with clumping of densely thickened loops in the absence of infiltration of the mesenteric fat. This patient has Crohn disease, which is more consistent with this white attenuation pattern of bowel wall thickening.
  - *Primary:* Without an obvious underlying cause (20%), this could be a consideration.

### ■ Essential Facts

- Acute mesenteric ischemia (AMI) may result from either arterial or venous obstruction.
- The attenuation pattern of diffusely dense bowel wall thickening seen in this case can occur with inflammatory bowel disease and vascular pathology.
- Symptomatic venous thrombosis typically involves the SMV rather than the inferior mesenteric vein, which drains a smaller distribution of bowel and has richer systemic (hemorrhoidal) and mesenteric collateral pathways.
- Causes of SMV thrombosis include hypercoagulable states, polycythemia, extrinsic compression or invasion by tumor, prior abdominal surgery, hypercoagulable states, portal vein thrombosis, cirrhosis and abdominal infection, fibrosis, or inflammation, as in this case.

- Clinical presentation of SMV thrombosis is more gradual than that of acute arterial thrombosis, increasing over days to months and ranging from mild abdominal discomfort to intense abdominal pain, nausea, vomiting, and fever (endotoxemia).
- Acute SMV thrombosis is onset within 4 months.
- Imaging findings depend on progression through a physiologic cascade:
  - Venous obstruction causes mesenteric infiltration and SB wall thickening due to edema. The more typical CT appearance of venous obstruction and small-bowel edema is the "water halo" or "target" sign of hypodense submucosa surrounded by hyperdense mucosa and muscularis.
  - Marked SB wall thickening due to venous hypertension may lead to arterial vasoconstriction.
  - Necrotic bowel may result, indicated by pneumatosis, mesenteric venous gas, and pneumatosis due to rupture.
- Prognosis with more rapid treatment is excellent, with a published mortality rate < 10%.
- Treatment is anticoagulation (sole treatment in many cases) and may progress to surgical thrombectomy and resection of infarcted bowel.

### ✓ Pearls & ✕ Pitfalls

- ✓ AMI may result from nonocclusive mesenteric ischemia (diffusely diminished splanchnic perfusion) or occlusive mesenteric ischemia.
- ✓ AMI usually results from embolism from a cardiac source or thrombosis of an atherosclerotic lesion.
- ✓ Bowel wall necrosis is uncommon in venous thrombosis but common in arterial thrombosis, often occurring within 12 hours.

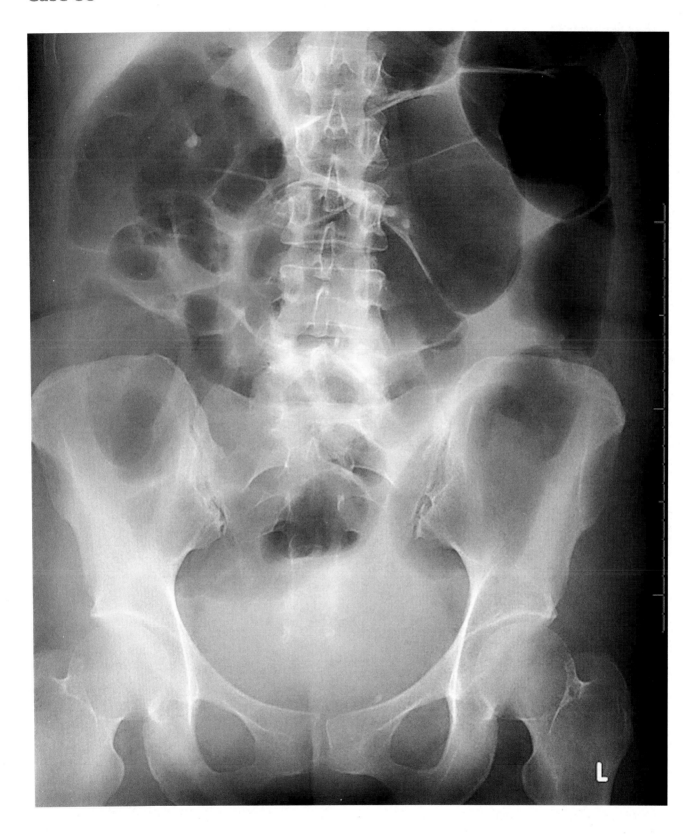

## Clinical Presentation

A 44-year-old woman presents with abdominal pain and distension.

### ◼ Imaging Findings

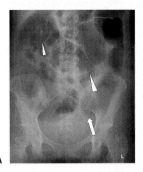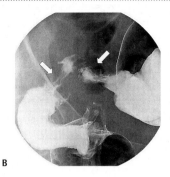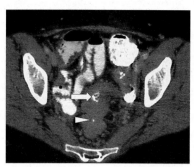

**(A)** Abdominal radiograph shows colonic dilatation (*large arrowhead*) terminating in the pelvis (*arrow*) and multiple air-filled ileal loops that are abnormal in caliber (*small arrowhead*). **(B)** Single-contrast barium enema shows an irregularly marginated stricture (*arrows*) of the rectosigmoid colon. **(C)** Pelvic computed tomography (CT) shows marked attenuation of the rectal lumen (*arrow*) leading to a critical stenosis (*arrowhead*) due to a circumferential infiltrating soft-tissue mass.

### ◼ Differential Diagnosis

- ***Rectosigmoid carcinoma:*** This is the most worrisome diagnosis and should be at the top of the list for distal colonic obstruction.
- *Intraluminal material:* Impacted feces or foreign bodies may cause distal obstruction. Fecal impaction is typically bubbly, but not always.
- *Inflammation or infection:* A third possibility, this can cause complete obstruction. Consider diverticulitis, inflammatory bowel disease, and proctocolitis due to lymphogranuloma venereum or tuberculosis.
- *Extrinsic causes:* These include pelvic tumor, abscess, adhesions, and bladder distension and are also worthy of consideration.
- *Inguinal hernia:* This can cause sigmoid obstruction.

### ◼ Essential Facts

- This case reviews the nonspecific radiographic finding of distal colonic obstruction. Paradoxically, distal colonic obstruction tends to cause maximal colonic distension in the cecum and more proximal colon.
- Colonic diameter of 6 cm (and cecal diameter of 10 cm) heralds impending rupture.
- Most neoplasms causing colonic obstruction occur in the rectosigmoid colon, but neoplasms occur about equally within the right and left colon.
- Colorectal carcinoma can occur as an infiltrating, annular mass ("apple-core"), as in this case, a polypoid mass, or an ulcerated mural mass.
- Competency of the ileocecal valve determines the bowel gas pattern on abdominal radiographs of colonic obstruction.
  - Competent: no small-bowel dilatation
  - Incompetent: small-bowel dilatation
- CT findings suggesting neoplasm over non-neoplastic causes include an exophytic mass with irregular borders, a spiculated mass obliterating pericolonic fat planes, invasion of adjacent organs, enlarged lymph nodes, and distal metastases. Bowel wall thickening is otherwise nonspecific.

- Staging (TNM):
  - T1: submucosa
  - T2: muscularis mucosae
  - T3: transmural
  - T4: invades adjacent organs/visceral peritoneum
  - N: positive nodes
  - M: distant metastases

### ◼ Other Imaging Findings

- Ultrasound (transrectal) provides an accurate staging of rectal carcinoma by assessing the depth of penetration of the mass into the bowel wall.

### ✓ Pearls & ✗ Pitfalls

✓ Intussusception causing colonic obstruction has a neoplastic lead point in the majority of cases but more commonly occurs in the ascending colon rather than in the rectosigmoid.

✓ Sigmoid volvulus is unlikely in this case as the classic signs such as the "coffee bean" sign and double loop obstruction are not present.

✗ Obstruction of the ileocecal valve by a markedly distended cecum may cause a pattern of dilated small and large bowel in cases of colonic obstruction, suggesting a generalized ileus and confusing the picture.

✗ Toxic megacolon is a clinical diagnosis based on colonic distension in the setting of an increased sedimentation rate, fever, leukocytosis, anemia, and bloody diarrhea.

✗ Pneumatosis, pneumoperitoneum, portal venous gas, and toxic megacolon are contraindications for barium enema.

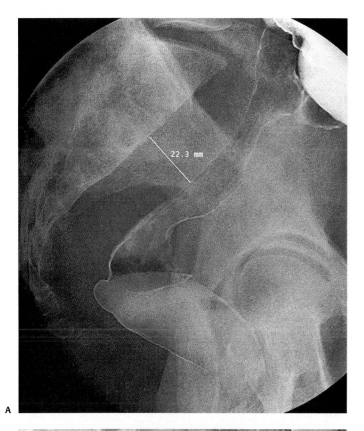

A

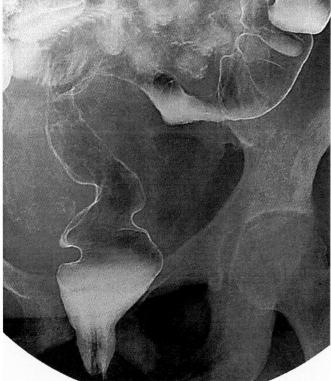

B

## ■ Clinical Presentation

A 47-year-old woman with breast cancer and a history of cord compression presents with pelvic cramping.

### ■ Imaging Findings

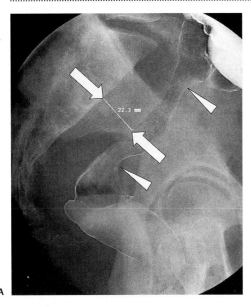
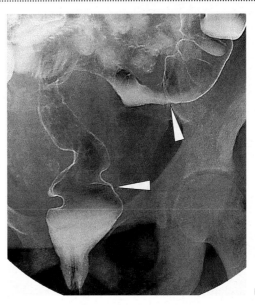

**(A)** Lateral projection during a double-contrast barium enema shows widening of the presacral space (*arrows*), effacement and narrowing of a long segment of rectosigmoid colon (*arrowheads*), and marked, diffuse sclerosis of the bones, consistent with metastatic disease from the known breast cancer. **(B)** Frontal projection shows persistence of the rectosigmoid stenosis (*arrowheads*) and an irregular mucosal pattern of the affected segment.

### ■ Differential Diagnosis

- **Radiation colitis:** This is the most likely diagnosis, caused by previous treatment of the patient's metastatic bone disease, given the long-segment colonic stricture, the mucosal effacement and irregularity, as well as the clinical history.
- *Rectosigmoid inflammation from inflammatory bowel disease:* This can result in focal stricture formation with mucosal effacement, particularly with Crohn disease.
- *Infectious colitis:* This can cause similar findings. Proctitis can be caused by gonococcal and herpes infections as well as lymphogranuloma venereum.
- *Benign encasement of the rectosigmoid:* This is another option caused by pelvic tumor, fat (pelvic lipomatosis), or blood (traumatic hematoma) that can produce stricturing and widening of the presacral space.

### ■ Essential Facts

- This case reviews the differential possibilities for strictures involving a long segment of colon as well as for widening of the presacral space. The differential diagnoses for these two findings overlap considerably.

- Radiation enteritis is endarteritis obliterans resulting in enteric ischemia due to radiation therapy. Chronic changes can cause focal narrowing and effacement of bowel segments in the radiation portal. Involvement of the rectum can cause widening of the presacral space.
- Chronically ischemic bowel can cause segmental colonic narrowing, but this entity rarely involves the rectum because of its rich collateral blood supply from inferior mesenteric and internal iliac arterial branches.

### ✓ Pearls & ✗ Pitfalls

- ✓ Presacral space is typically < 2 cm wide.
- ✓ Intrinsic processes such as rectosigmoid infection or inflammation can lead to chronic segmental narrowing with widening of the presacral space. Consider inflammatory bowel diseases, infectious proctitis/colitis, and infiltration by adenocarcinoma or lymphoma.
- ✓ Extrinsic processes can cause segmental narrowing with widening of the presacral space.
- ✓ Consider pelvic lipomatosis, pelvic tumors, pericolonic abscesses, and pelvic hematoma.

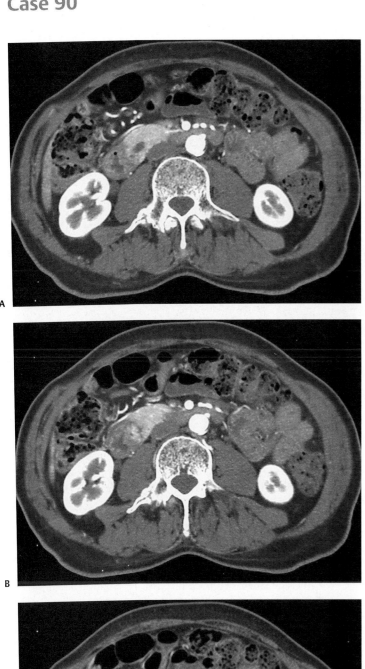

A

B

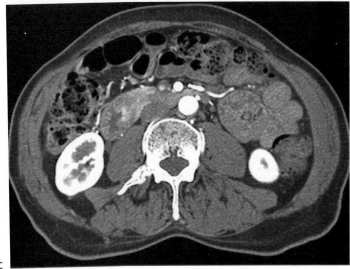

C

## Clinical Presentation

A 55-year-old man presents with jaundice.

### ■ Imaging Findings

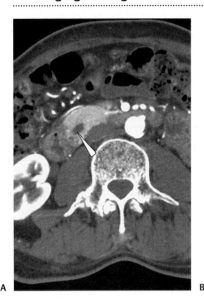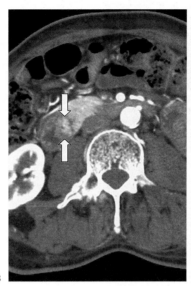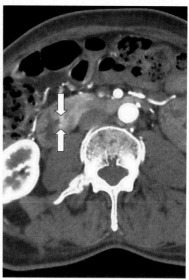

A  B  C

**(A)** Contrast-enhanced computed tomography (CT) in the arterial phase shows a prominent common bile duct (CBD; *arrowhead*). **(B,C)** Adjacent images show early enhancement of an enlarged papilla (*arrows*), which measures 2 cm in diameter.

### ■ Differential Diagnosis

- ***Ampullary carcinoma:*** This is the most likely diagnosis, given the papillary enlargement and early enhancement.
- *Cholangiocarcinoma:* This is a consideration as it may have identical features.
- *Duodenal tumors:* An adenoma or adenocarcinoma may be periampullary in location.

### ■ Essential Facts

- The papilla of Vater normally drains both the CBD and the main pancreatic duct (PD). The enhancement pattern of the papilla is normally similar to that of the adjacent CBD.
- Improvements in helical CT scanners have resulted in improved detection of subtle periampullary neoplasms, a term describing any tumor affecting this region (typically adenocarcinoma of the ampulla, bile duct, pancreas, or duodenum).
- When encountering a mass in the medial aspect of the second portion of the duodenum on CT, try to establish an association with the CBD and PD to classify it as a periampullary mass.
- Circumferential, enhancing periampullary masses most likely represent ampullary carcinoma or cholangiocarcinoma.

### ■ Other Imaging Findings

- Upper gastrointestinal barium studies showing papillary enlargement are nonspecific, but enlargement of the papilla beyond 1.5 cm in any dimension should be considered abnormal and further investigated by endoscopy or CT.

### ✓ Pearls & ✗ Pitfalls

✓ Lesions simulating papillary masses on imaging studies include small, ectopic pancreatic rests (similar bull's-eye appearance on barium study), duodenal polyps, and submucosal masses such as leiomyomas and gastrointestinal stromal tumors.

✓ Papillary edema may simulate a mass and be caused by papillitis, pancreatitis, or a stone impacted at the papilla.

✓ Pancreatic carcinoma is most commonly located in the pancreatic head and may be small and barely detectable by indirect signs of a bulging papilla as well as dilatation of the CBD and PD. Unlike this case, this entity is usually hypodense rather than brightly enhancing.

✗ Masses detected on the medial aspect of the second portion of the duodenum are not always periampullary neoplasms.

✗ Anomalous location of the papilla of Vater at the third portion of the duodenum may occur.

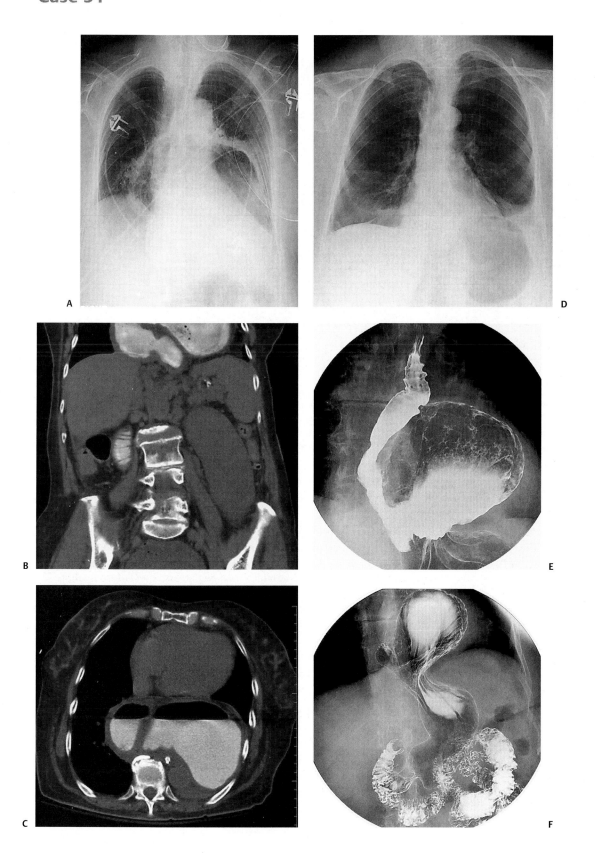

A

D

B

E

C

F

## Clinical Presentation

For the following two patients with midepigastric pain, what is the differential diagnosis for the radiographic findings?
What are the diagnosis and clinical significance in each case?

### ◼ Imaging Findings

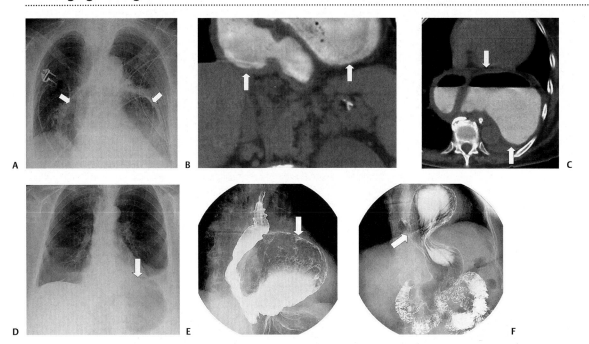

**(A)** Radiograph of the first patient shows an air-filled structure (*arrows*) in the chest. **(B)** Coronal computed tomography (CT) with oral contrast shows an intrathoracic stomach (*arrows*). Barium within the stomach indicates absence of complete volvulus, although partial organoaxial volvulus is present (see below). **(C)** Axial CT shows a nasogastric (NG) tube passing posterior to the stomach (*arrows*) toward the gastroesophageal junction (GEJ). **(D)** Radiograph of the second patient shows a large, air-filled structure in the left upper quadrant/chest (*arrow*). **(E)** Barium study shows near-normal position of the GEJ and a large paraesophageal hernia (*arrow*). **(F)** Additional image shows normal GEJ position.

### ◼ Differential Diagnosis

- **_Paraesophageal hiatal hernia:_** This is strongly indicated in both cases by verification of the GEJ at or near its normal subdiaphragmatic position despite all or a portion of the stomach being herniated upward through the diaphragmatic hiatus. Intrathoracic stomach is a form of paraesophageal hiatal hernia.
- *Diaphragmatic eventration:* This is a second choice, although it may be difficult to distinguish from hiatal hernia in some cases.
- *Gastric pull-up:* This is usually distinguishable by a gastroesophageal anastomosis high in the thorax.

### ◼ Essential Facts

- Paraesophageal hiatal hernia occurs when some portion of the stomach passes up through the diaphragmatic hiatus but the GEJ remains fixed at or near its normal position. All or part of the stomach may be in the thorax.
- Rolling hiatal hernia describes an intrathoracic position of only part of the stomach despite a subdiaphragmatic position of the GEJ.
  - Barium study shows the herniated portion anterior to the esophagus despite a normally positioned GEJ.
  - It is difficult or impossible to reduce in many cases and may be associated with ischemic volvulus, incarceration, or perforation.

- Intrathoracic stomach describes an intrathoracic position of the stomach despite the GEJ residing at or near its normal position.
  - Barium study shows the GEJ at or near its normal position.
  - Gastric volvulus may be present: mesenteroaxial, organoaxial, or both.
- Congenitally short esophagus may look like a gastric pull-up with the GEJ high in the chest.
- Chronic achalasia is an unlikely choice but can result in marked distension of the esophagus in the chest with the GEJ remaining subdiaphragmatic.

### ◼ Other Imaging Findings

- CT may show pneumatosis, mural thickening, and free air due to strangulation or perforation.
- Barium study may show absent passage of barium into the stomach in cases of gastric volvulus.

### ✓ Pearls & ✗ Pitfalls

- ✓ For complete volvulus (> 180 degrees), there is no passage of barium or NG tube into the stomach.

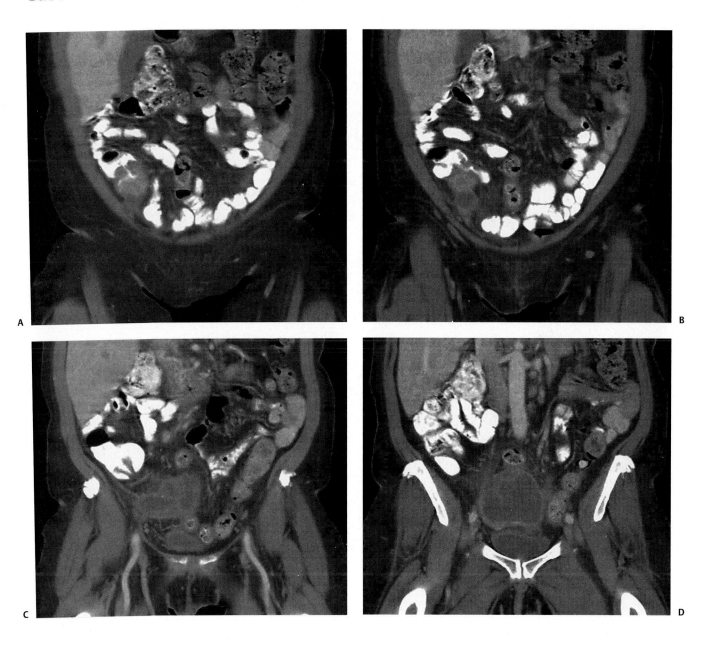

## Clinical Presentation

A 75-year-old woman presents with pelvic pain and is found to have fever and leukocytosis.

### ■ Imaging Findings

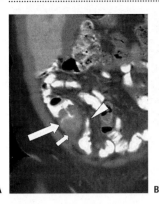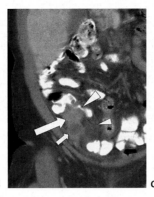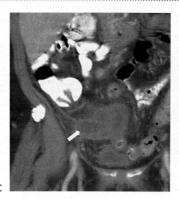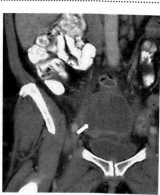

A                                 B                               C                               D

**(A)** Coronal reformatted infused computed tomography shows a mass (*large arrow*) in the cecum with adjacent mural thickening. A fluid-density structure (*small arrow*) abutting this mass may represent the base of a dilated appendix. The barium-filled terminal ileum is annotated (*arrowhead*). **(B)** More posterior image shows the mass (*large arrow*), the base of the appendix (*small arrow*), the ileocecal valve (*large arrowhead*), and pericecal fat stranding (*small arrowhead*). **(C)** More posterior image shows the dilated appendix (*arrow*). **(D)** More posterior image shows a large, septated, thick-walled fluid collection (*arrow*) representing a pelvic abscess due to ruptured appendicitis.

### ■ Differential Diagnosis

- ***Cecal carcinoma causing appendicitis:*** This is the most likely diagnosis for a cecal mass with an adjacent fluid collection suspicious for ruptured appendicitis.
- *Appendiceal adenocarcinoma:* This can occur at the base of the appendix, causing obstruction and appendicitis.
- *Carcinoid:* This is less likely. It most commonly affects the appendix and small bowel. However, in the appendix, carcinoid is usually benign.

### ■ Essential Facts

- When findings suggest appendicitis, consider any cause of appendiceal obstruction to avoid missing a grave diagnosis, such as carcinoma.
- Causes of appendiceal obstruction include lymphoid hyperplasia, appendicolith, tumor, and inflammatory bowel disease (particularly Crohn disease).
- Infection or inflammation of the colon may be indistinguishable from colon carcinoma in up to 10% of cases.
- Signs of neoplasm are all illustrated in this case and include more marked wall thickening, a polypoid mass, annular infiltration, and less pericolonic infiltration compared with infectious or inflammatory etiologies.

### ✓ Pearls & ✗ Pitfalls

- ✓ Pelvic appendicitis and tubo-ovarian abscess may be indistinguishable. In women older than 60 years, both conditions have a higher risk for an underlying malignant cause.
- ✓ Lymphoma may originate from the appendix or terminal ileum and infiltrate the cecal wall (coned cecum). Lymphoma may mimic or, less commonly, cause appendicitis.
- ✓ Crohn disease can cause cecal wall thickening and appendicitis in up to 25% of cases. Look for involvement of the terminal ileum.

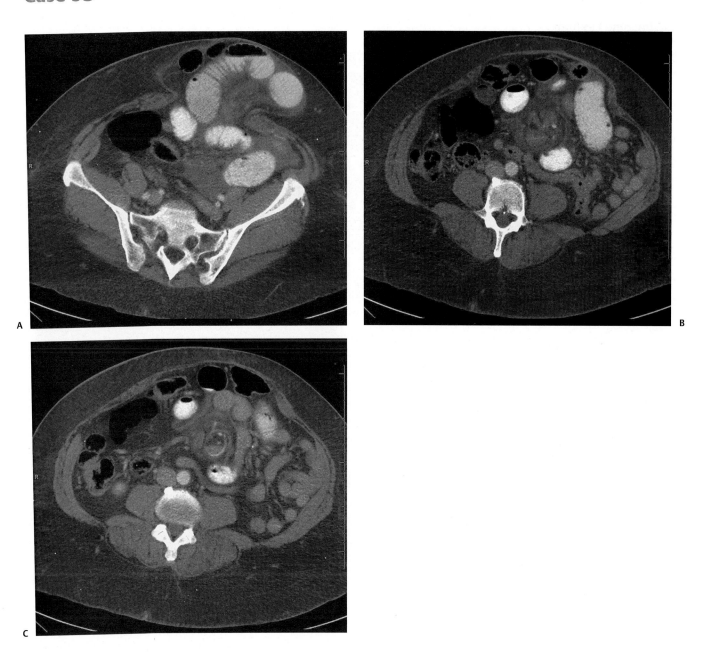

## Clinical Presentation

A 62-year-old woman presents with abdominal pain and distension.

## ■ Imaging Findings

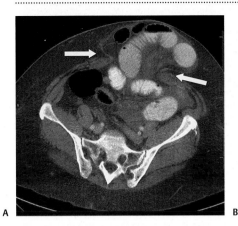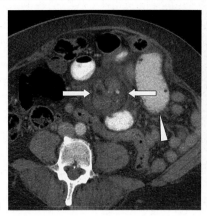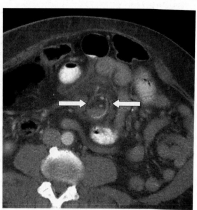

**(A)** Contrast-enhanced computed tomography (CT) shows a wide-mouthed ventral hernia (*arrows*) containing both colon and small bowel. There is associated small-bowel dilatation, adjacent fat stranding, and a small amount of ascites. **(B)** Abdominal CT shows a rounded focus (*arrows*) containing small bowel, mesenteric fat, and mesenteric vessels. There is an adjacent, dilated small-bowel loop (*arrowhead*). **(C)** Image obtained at the root of the mesentery shows whirling mesenteric vessels, consistent with mesenteric volvulus (*arrows*).

## ■ Differential Diagnosis

- ***Mesenteric volvulus with ventral hernia:*** This is the only diagnosis, given the characteristic finding of whirling mesenteric vessels associated with dilated small bowel located within an external hernia.

## ■ Essential Facts

- Mesenteric volvulus is abnormal rotation of the mesentery, placing the patient at risk for bowel obstruction and ischemia.
- It is associated with malrotation and prior abdominal surgery and commonly occurs within internal or external hernias, as in this case.
- Currently, this patient has a partial small-bowel obstruction as contrast fills the dilated loops. However, to some degree, the following are present:
  - Closed loop obstruction: a segment of bowel obstructs at both ends and becomes fluid-filled and distended.
  - Strangulation of herniated bowel: Mechanical obstruction with interrupted blood flow, placing the patient at risk for necrosis. Imaging findings include bowel wall thickening, distension of the bowel lumen by fluid, adjacent fat stranding from edema, and exudate and ascites.
- Necrosis would be the final stage of bowel injury by pneumatosis, pneumoperitoneum from perforation, and portal or mesenteric venous gas.

## ✓ Pearls & ✗ Pitfalls

- ✓ Closed-loop obstructions can also be due to adhesions and masses.
- ✗ Failure to diagnose mesenteric volvulus or closed loop small-bowel obstruction may lead to the cascading development of torsion of venous outflow, luminal distension by fluid due to increased hydrostatic pressure, mural edema and hemorrhage, compromised arterial inflow, and infarction.

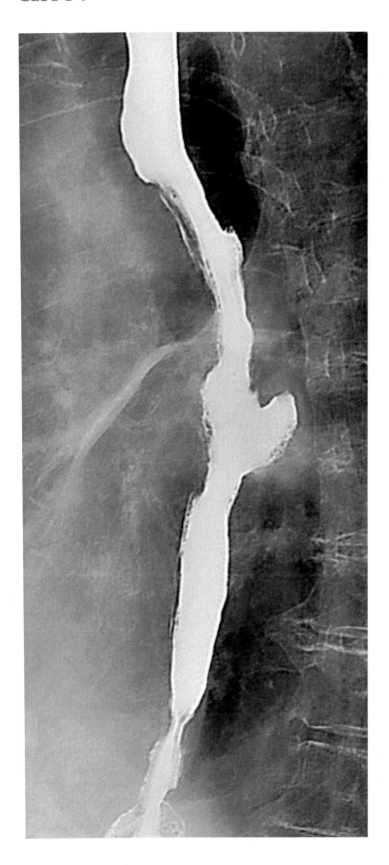

## ■ Clinical Presentation

A 69-year-old man has dysphagia.

■ **Imaging Findings**

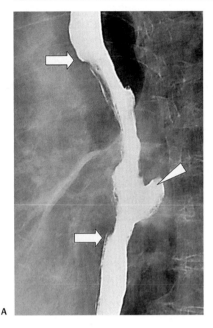

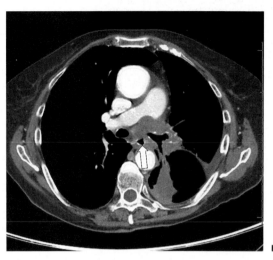

A                                                                                                                    B

**(A)** Single-contrast barium study shows a long, irregularly marginated midesophageal stricture (*arrows*). A focal, posterolateral outpouching (*arrowhead*) of contrast is also visible. **(B)** Contrast-enhanced computed tomography (CT) shows a soft-tissue mass infiltrating the mediastinum at the level of the carina and narrowing the esophageal lumen (*arrow*).

■ **Differential Diagnosis**

- ***Malignant ulcer:*** This is the top diagnosis, given the associated, irregularly marginated stricture in the mid-esophagus, highly suspicious for a malignant stricture. The CT image confirms the malignant etiology.
- *Traction diverticulum:* This can have a similar appearance.

■ **Essential Facts**

- This patient previously underwent resection of lung cancer and has direct invasion of the esophagus by malignant mediastinal lymphadenopathy.
- Malignant ulcer and stricture of the esophagus:
  - May occur via direct invasion by an adjacent malignancy
  - Sources at the midesophageal level include metastatic lymphadenopathy from breast or lung carcinoma or direct invasion by mediastinal malignancies, such as lymphoma.
  - Occurrence at the distal esophageal level is typically due to esophageal extension of gastric adenocarcinoma.
- Traction diverticula of the esophagus:
  - Commonly midthoracic, but may occur throughout the esophagus
  - Propensity for midthoracic location is due to a relationship to prior inflammation of hilar and mediastinal adenopathy.
  - Variety of shapes and sizes

✓ **Pearls & ✗ Pitfalls**

- ✓ Hematogenous metastases to the esophagus are uncommon but may occur with the greatest frequency in patients with breast cancer or malignant melanoma.
- ✗ Malignant invasion of the esophagus and mediastinum may result in a bronchoesophageal fistula. Use of barium contrast over water-soluble contrast is recommended if this entity is suspected.

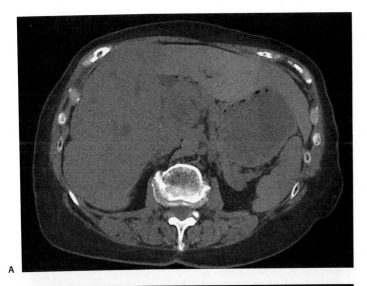

**A**

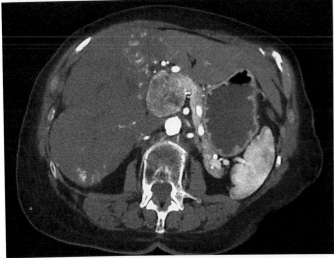

**B**

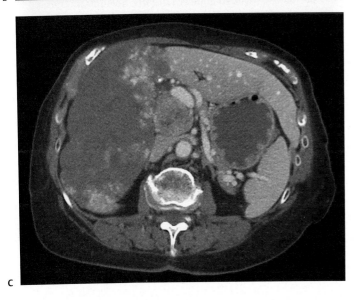

**C**

## ▨ Clinical Presentation

A 59-year-old man presents with abdominal pain and weight loss.

## ■ Imaging Findings

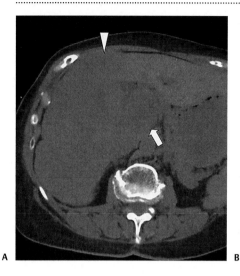
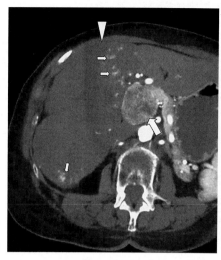
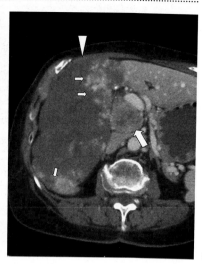

A                                                    B                                                    C

**(A)** Noninfused computed tomography (CT) shows a large, hypodense, uncalcified mass (*arrowhead*) replacing most of the right lobe of the liver. In addition, there is a large, uncalcified mass (*arrow*) occupying and expanding the porta hepatis. **(B)** Arterial-phase contrast-enhanced CT shows focal areas of contrast pooling (*small arrows*) in the periphery of the large hepatic mass (*arrowhead*). The mass in the porta hepatis (*large arrow*) occupies the location of the pancreatic head and heterogeneously enhances with pancreatic tissue. The pancreatic body and tail appear atrophied. **(C)** Venous-phase imaging shows further patchy peripheral enhancement (*small arrows*) of the large hepatic mass (*arrowhead*), and diminished enhancement of the tumor in the pancreatic head (*large arrow*) similar to that in the pancreatic body and tail.

## ■ Differential Diagnosis

- ***Primary pancreatic carcinoma and cavernous hemangioma of the liver:*** The patient's age, the presentation, and the location within the pancreatic head suggest pancreatic adenocarcinoma, which is the top diagnosis in this case. However, moderate arterial-phase enhancement is more suggestive of islet cell tumor or hypervascular metastasis.
- *Metastatic pancreatic lesion:* This is statistically less likely.
- *Microcystic adenoma of the pancreas:* This is worthy as a consideration, given the lack of invasion of adjacent organs and vessels, the well-circumscribed appearance, and the absence of lymphadenopathy or hepatic metastasis. A diffuse, multicystic appearance, a radiating central stellate scar, and punctate calcifications would support this diagnosis but are not clearly seen in this case.

## ■ Essential Facts

- The imaging features of this hepatic tumor are pathognomonic for a cavernous hemangioma: an uncalcified, low-density mass on noninfused imaging and peripheral enhancement on arterial-phase imaging that increases on the delayed phase. The mistake to avoid is missing the life-threatening pancreatic tumor!
- Pancreatic adenocarcinoma is a malignant tumor usually originating from duct cells and occurring after 55 years of age. The uncharacteristic enhancement in this case should prompt diagnostic consideration of a hypervascular lesion such as islet cell tumor or metastasis.

- Associations with pancreatic adenocarcinoma include smoking, a history of alcohol-related or hereditary pancreatitis, and diabetes.
- Clinical presentation may include the new onset of diabetes, jaundice, pain radiating to the back, and nonspecific symptoms of nausea and weight loss.
- CT findings suggesting adenocarcinoma are location in the pancreatic head (60%), centrally hypoattenuating necrosis, a dilated pancreatic duct, effaced peripancreatic fat planes, invaded adjacent organs, invaded or encased vessels, regional adenopathy, and distant metastasis.
- Primary adenocarcinoma may present as a small, barely detectable mass in the pancreatic head with enhancement similar to that of adjacent pancreatic parenchyma. Look for indirect findings of pancreatic duct obstruction or double-duct sign (obstruction of pancreatic and common bile ducts).

## ✓ Pearls & ✗ Pitfalls

- ✓ Islet cell tumors tend to present while small (< 2 cm) because of the secretion of functional hormones and tend to be hypervascular. However, a nonfunctional islet cell tumor may present as a large, heterogeneous mass with an appearance similar to this case.
- ✗ Most tumors of the pancreas are typically resected if focal, noninvasive, and symptomatic.
- ✗ Do not miss details suggesting an unresectable, malignant pancreatic adenocarcinoma, such as invaded adjacent organs, encased or invaded vessels, malignant ascites, and distant metastasis.

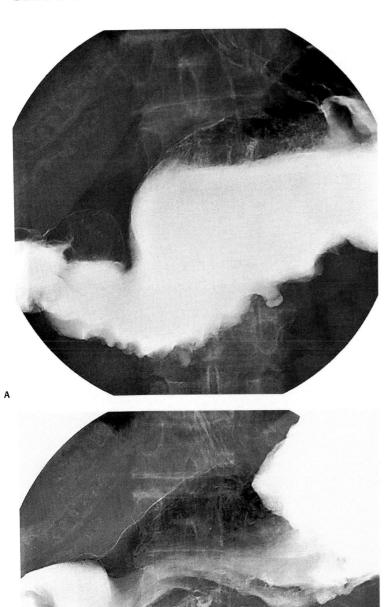

A

B

## Clinical Presentation

A 57-year-old woman presents with midepigastric pain, nausea, vomiting, and weight loss.

### ■ Imaging Findings

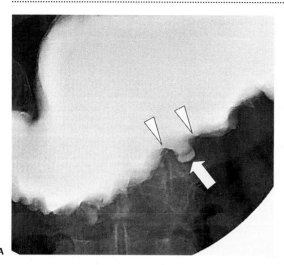
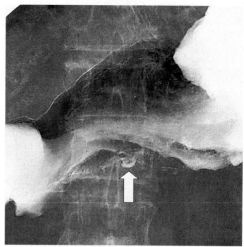

**(A)** Single-contrast study of the stomach shows a 1-cm ulcer crater (*arrow*) along the greater curvature surrounded by a nodular, circumferential mass (*arrowheads*). The ulcer crater appears intraluminal rather than extending beyond the confines of the gastric lumen. **(B)** Double-contrast study again shows the crater (*arrow*) surrounded by a circumferential mass. There are no radiating folds extending to the ulcer crater, and the adjacent gastric mucosa appears featureless. The nearby gastric rugae are markedly thickened.

### ■ Differential Diagnosis

- ***Malignant gastric ulcer:*** This is indicated by an ulcer crater projecting within the confines of the gastric lumen; a nodular, circumferential mass surrounding the crater; featureless regional mucosa; and gastric folds failing to extend to the crater.
- *Benign gastric ulcer:* This is far less likely, although markedly edematous folds surrounding a peptic ulcer can mimic the findings of a malignant ulcer.

### ■ Essential Facts

- The key to this case is not just identifying the ulcer, but also recognizing the imaging differences between the two principal types of gastric ulcer: a malignant gastric ulcer and a benign peptic ulcer.
- Malignant gastric ulcers result from ulcerations within tumors and:
  - Arise from several tumor types, including primary gastric adenocarcinoma, gastrointestinal stromal tumor, leiomyosarcoma, and metastasis.
  - May appear in locations atypical for peptic ulcers, such as the fundus (see below).
  - Typically project within the confines of the gastric lumen.
  - May be surrounded by irregular, nodular soft tissue and featureless mucosa with absent areae gastricae.
  - Lack barium-filled folds radiating to the edge of the crater.

- Gastric peptic ulcers:
  - Are usually located along the lesser curve or posterior wall of the body or antrum.
  - Usually project beyond the gastric lumen.
  - May be surrounded by a smooth rim of edematous folds (ulcer mound), prominent areae gastricae, and a radiolucent line (Hampton line) that separates the barium-filled crater from the barium-coated stomach wall.
  - May have barium-filled folds radiating directly to the edge of the ulcer crater.

### ✓ Pearls & ✗ Pitfalls

- ✓ Malignant tumors cause only 5% of gastric ulcers.
- ✓ Benign peptic ulcers more commonly (95%) occur in the duodenum rather than in the stomach.
- ✓ Large, benign tumors may ulcerate.
- ✗ Anterior wall gastric ulcers are less common and more difficult to detect. They appear as rings of barium coating the crater edge.
- ✗ Chronic scarring from peptic ulcers can mimic radiating folds of active ulcers or mural findings of malignancy.
- ✗ Endoscopy should be recommended if malignancy is suspected.

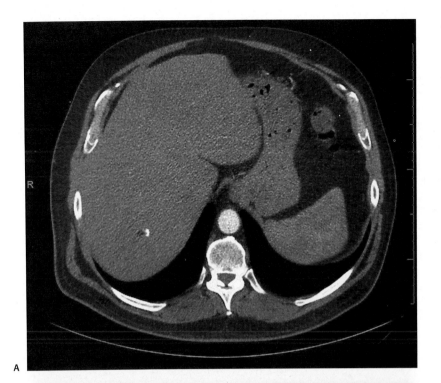

A

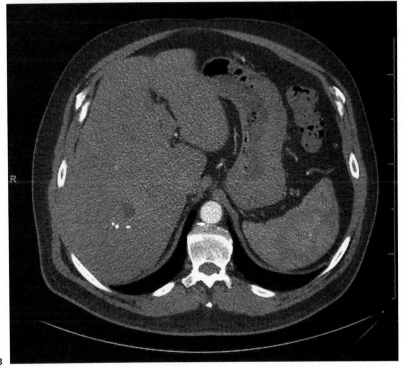

B

## ■ Clinical Presentation

A 50-year-old man presents for computed tomography work-up of a liver lesion noted on ultrasound.

### ■ Imaging Findings

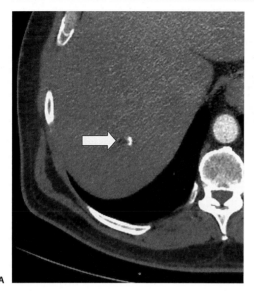 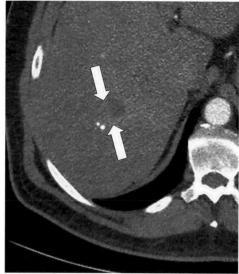

**(A)** Contrast-enhanced computed tomography (CT) in the arterial phase shows a focus of macroscopic fat within the right lobe of the liver with an adjacent dense calcification (*arrow*). **(B)** More caudal slice shows a heterogeneous soft-tissue mass (*arrows*) with peripheral dense calcifications.

### ■ Differential Diagnosis

- **Metastatic germ cell tumor:** This is the principal diagnostic consideration for a mass in the liver with patchy macroscopic fat, a soft-tissue component, and dense calcifications. The calcification in Figure A has the appearance of a tooth.
- *Liposarcoma:* Usually metastatic, this option belongs on the differential for macroscopic fat but is very rare in the liver. Calcification is uncommon.
- *Angiomyolipoma:* This rarely occurs in the liver and typically has a heterogeneous appearance due to enhancing soft-tissue components, ectatic arteries, and foci of macroscopic fat. Calcification is uncommon.

### ■ Essential Facts

- Germ cell tumor occurring in the liver may be a primary hepatic teratoma (exceedingly rare) or a germ cell metastasis from an extrahepatic malignancy (more common, but still rare). Characteristic heterogeneity may be a distinguishing feature and is caused by a combination of cells of ectodermal, endodermal, and mesodermal origin.
- Hepatocellular carcinoma (HCC) may contain patchy regions of macroscopic fat in 10 to 35% of cases.
  - HCC of chronic liver disease or cirrhosis rarely calcifies and is an unlikely explanation for the lesion in this case.
  - Fibrolamellar carcinoma commonly calcifies, but with a more amorphous appearance, unlike the toothlike appearance in this case.

- Hepatic adenoma may contain microscopic intracellular fat or focal patches of macroscopic fat that may be quite prominent, with an appearance similar to that of HCC (< 10% of adenomas have fat visible on CT). However, adenomas typically do not calcify.
- Other benign masses with macroscopic fat that rarely calcify include metastatic liposarcoma angiomyolipoma, myelolipoma, and lipoma.

### ■ Other Imaging Findings

- Magnetic resonance imaging is the best modality to identify fat within any tumor, evidenced by increased signal on T1, decreased signal on T2, and signal dropout on out-of-phase gradient-echo images compared with in-phase images (chemical shift).

### ✓ Pearls & ✗ Pitfalls

- ✓ Macroscopic fat occurs in both benign and malignant masses and is therefore a nonspecific finding.
- ✓ Look for associated features suspicious for malignancy, such as rapid growth, enhancing soft-tissue components, and vascular invasion.

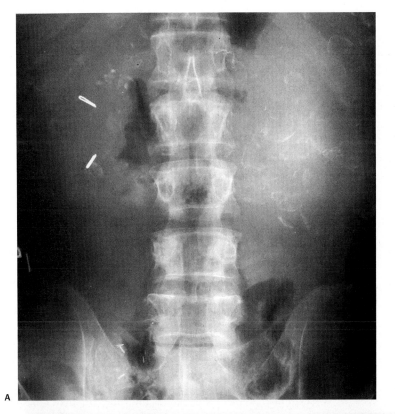

A

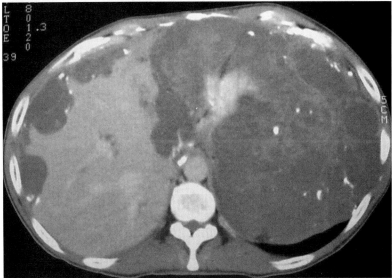

B

## ▓ Clinical Presentation

A 63-year-old woman presents with abdominal distension and pain.

## ◼ Imaging Findings

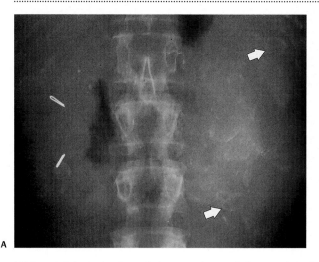
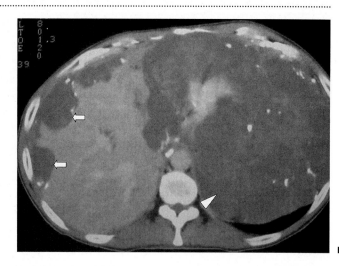

**(A)** Frontal abdominal radiograph shows curvilinear calcifications throughout the abdomen (*arrows*). **(B)** Contrast-enhanced computed tomography in the venous phase shows scalloping of the liver margin (*arrows*) and nonenhancing, low-density material throughout the abdomen (*arrowhead*) with septations and scattered calcifications.

## ◼ Differential Diagnosis

- **Pseudomyxoma peritonei:** This is the top diagnosis. Scattered, diffuse, curvilinear calcifications within diffuse, septated, low-density material throughout the abdomen are highly suggestive of this entity.
- *Disseminated mucinous carcinomatosis:* This is similar and is caused by mucinous ascites produced by a high-grade mucin-producing carcinoma.
- *Mesothelioma:* This is a possibility. It may be either cystic malignant or benign multicystic.

## ◼ Essential Facts

- Pseudomyxoma peritonei is rupture of mucinous adenocarcinoma or peritoneal carcinomatosis leading to gradual filling of the peritoneum with gelatinous material.
- Offending neoplasms include ovarian mucinous cystadenocarcinoma (most commonly), mucinous adenocarcinoma of the appendix, and rarely adenocarcinoma of the stomach and colon and mucinous tumors of the pancreas.
- Clinical presentation varies but typically includes increasing abdominal girth with or without associated hernia.
- Imaging studies show scalloping of the liver, omental caking, and displacement of bowel and mesenteric vessels by the gelatinous, septate material.

- Treatment consists of surgical debulking and intraperitoneal chemotherapy.
- Other diagnostic considerations:
  - Lymphangioma may appear as multiple confluent cysts within the abdomen, omentum, or mesentery containing protein-rich chylous fluid.
  - Pyogenic peritonitis rarely has this appearance, but the clinical picture would be severe abdominal pain and sepsis.

## ◼ Other Imaging Findings

- Abdominal radiography may show the curvilinear calcifications seen in this case. This is a rare but nearly pathognomonic finding.

## ✓ Pearls & ✗ Pitfalls

- ✓ Think of this entity in patients with massive, septated ascites and liver scalloping.
- ✓ Echinococcal cysts throughout the abdomen may have this appearance, although this presentation is extremely rare.

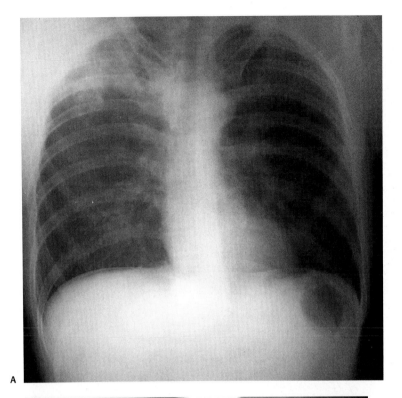

A

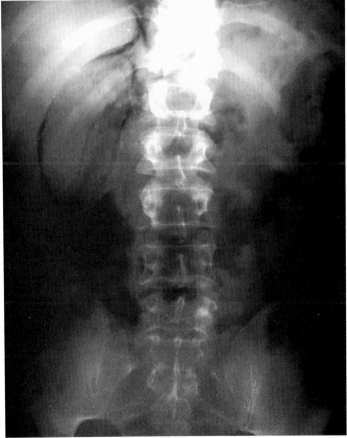

B

## ▧ Clinical Presentation

..............................................................................................................................

A 25-year-old man is found unconscious on the ground and taken to the emergency department.

### ■ Imaging Findings

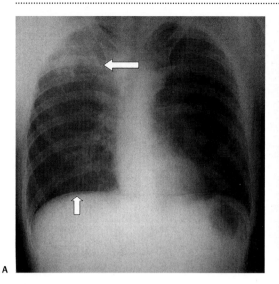
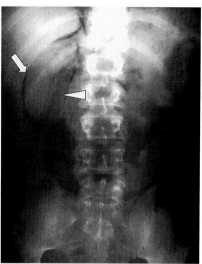

**(A)** Upright abdominal radiograph shows pneumoperitoneum manifesting as a thin rim of subdiaphragmatic gas (*small arrow*). A presumed pulmonary contusion is visible (*large arrow*). **(B)** Abdominal radiograph shows a bubbly gas collection in the perirenal space (*arrowhead*), extending along the inferior margin of the liver (*arrow*).

### ■ Differential Diagnosis

- ***Traumatic duodenal rupture:*** This is the most likely diagnosis, given the combination of retroperitoneal gas and pneumoperitoneum. The presumed pulmonary contusion supports the diagnosis by providing evidence of trauma.
- *Duodenal rupture from peptic ulcer disease or neoplasm:* This can produce identical findings, but the pulmonary finding makes this less likely (see also below).
- *Renal or perirenal abscess:* This may outline the kidney in a manner demonstrated by the abdominal radiograph in this case. However, the pneumoperitoneum makes this diagnosis least likely.

### ■ Essential Facts

- Retroperitoneal gas is usually caused by a ruptured duodenum or rectum. The ascending and descending segments of the colon are also retroperitoneal structures and may be the source of retroperitoneal gas in some cases.
- Sources of retroperitoneal gas include pneumatosis intestinalis of the colon or duodenum from trauma, ischemia, or infection, and gas-containing abscesses originating from the colon (e.g., diverticulitis, iatrogenic injury from colonoscopy), pancreas (pancreatic abscess or infected pseudocyst), or urinary tract.
- Radiographic findings of retroperitoneal gas are easiest to detect on the right side as gas dissects along the inferior margin of the liver, streaks along the psoas muscle, and outlines the kidney.
- Rupture of the duodenum results from trauma, iatrogenic injury (endoscopy), peptic ulcer disease, and malignancy.

- Lymphomatous infiltration of the small bowel is associated with a high incidence of rupture (up to 40%), especially during treatment with chemotherapy.
- As this case illustrates, the duodenum is a fixed, retroperitoneal structure (except for the bulb) coursing anteriorly across the spinal column; as a result, it absorbs most of the force of impact during major trauma.
- Radiographic findings of duodenal trauma may include free retroperitoneal gas, duodenal pneumatosis intestinalis, pneumoperitoneum, and pneumomediastinum.

### ■ Other Imaging Findings

- Computed tomography is performed in all patients with abnormal gas detected by radiography.

### ✓ Pearls & ✗ Pitfalls

- ✓ Retroperitoneal gas remains fixed in position during a comparison of supine and lateral decubitus abdominal radiographs.
- ✓ Whenever retroperitoneal gas is observed, look for other signs of trauma, such as pulmonary contusions and fractures of the ribs and spine.
- ✗ Small foci of extraluminal gas on abdominal radiographs can be mistaken for intraluminal bowel gas.
- ✗ Evidence of extraluminal gas includes bubbly collections that fail to coalesce into a single gas pocket on successive radiographs, and fixed collections that fail to move when the patient changes position (supine to prone or lateral decubitus position).

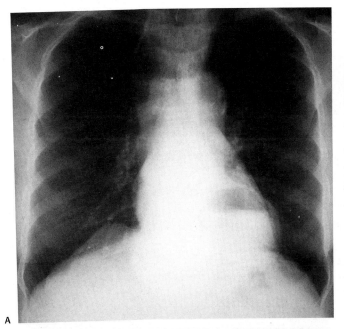

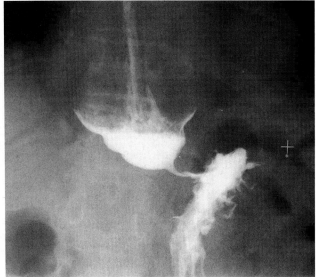

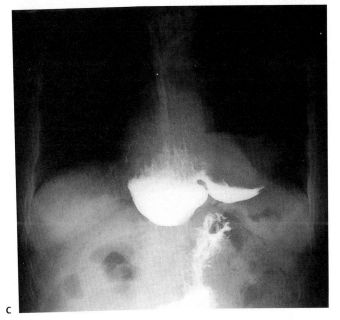

## ■ Clinical Presentation

A 71-year-old man presents with halitosis.

### ■ Imaging Findings

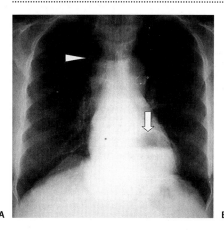 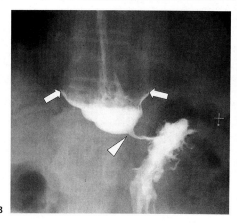 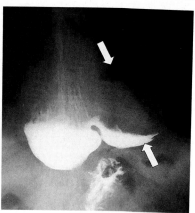

A     B     C

**(A)** Frontal chest radiograph shows a large, air-filled structure extending from the upper to the lower chest (*arrowhead*) and a large air-fluid level in the retrocardiac left lower chest (*arrow*). **(B)** Barium study shows a markedly dilated esophagus, or "megaesophagus" (*arrows*), a "rat tail" deformity of the lower esophageal sphincter (*arrowhead*), and slow passage of contrast into the stomach. **(C)** Delayed image shows a large, round paraesophageal collection containing an air-fluid level and dependent layering of barium (*arrows*).

### ■ Differential Diagnosis

- ***Achalasia with epiphrenic diverticulum:*** This is the top choice, given the megaesophagus, the rat tail stricture of the distal esophagus, and an epiphrenic saccular outpouching from the esophagus.
- *Secondary achalasia and pseudoachalasia:* These are possible explanations for a strictured lower esophageal sphincter in this configuration

### ■ Essential Facts

- Achalasia with epiphrenic diverticulum is an unusual combination, and the challenge of this case is identifying these two entities and understanding the reason for their occasional association (see "Pearls & Pitfalls").
- This case illustrates the classic features of achalasia, including retention of barium and debris within an atonic esophagus, narrowing of the lower esophageal sphincter (LES) in a "rat tail" or "bird's beak" configuration, and marked dilatation of the entire esophageal lumen.
- This case also illustrates the classic features of an epiphrenic diverticulum, including a large, well-circumscribed, saccular structure containing an air-fluid level on chest radiograph that fills with barium on esophagogram.
- Paraesophageal hernia, hiatal hernia, diaphragmatic eventration, gastric pull-up, achalasia, bronchial or esophageal rupture, and mediastinal abscess are all diagnostic options for a large air-fluid level on chest radiography.

### ■ Other Imaging Findings

- Esophagogram would demonstrate the dysmotility of achalasia, including aperistalsis of the entire esophagus (typically progresses from the proximal to the distal esophagus), the intermittent passage of barium through the narrowed LES when esophageal pressure is transiently sufficient (and when carbonation is ingested), and relaxation of the LES when amyl nitrate is inhaled.

### ✓ Pearls & ✗ Pitfalls

- ✓ The constant intraluminal pressure of achalasia may result in pulsion diverticula. In this case:
  - Unlike in paraesophageal hernia, diaphragmatic eventration, and gastric pull-up, barium in the stomach does not communicate directly with the paraesophageal sac.
  - Unlike in hiatal hernia or gastric pull-up, the gastroesophageal junction is in its normal location below the diaphragm.
  - Unlike in esophageal rupture and mediastinal abscess, the air-filled paraesophageal sac is round and well circumscribed.
- ✗ Do not miss life-threatening considerations for an air-fluid level on chest radiography, such as esophageal rupture and mediastinal abscess.
- ✗ For esophageal or bronchial perforation, look for pneumomediastinum, subcutaneous emphysema, and hydro(pneumo)thorax.
- ✗ Avoid "satisfaction-of-search" phenomenon when a single large finding is discovered.

## Case 1

Bennett GL, Rusinek H, Lisi V, et al. CT findings in acute gangrenous cholecystitis. AJR Am J Roentgenol 2002;178(2):275–281

## Case 2

Gupta A, Stuhlfaut JW, Fleming KW, Lucey BC, Soto JA. Blunt trauma of the pancreas and biliary tract: a multimodality imaging approach to diagnosis. Radiographics 2004;24(5):1381–1395

## Case 3

Casillas VJ, Amendola MA, Gascue A, Pinnar N, Levi JU, Perez JM. Imaging of nontraumatic hemorrhagic hepatic lesions. Radiographics 2000;20(2):367–378

## Case 4

Ghai S, Pattison J, Ghai S, O'Malley ME, Khalili K, Stephens M. Primary gastrointestinal lymphoma: spectrum of imaging findings with pathologic correlation. Radiographics 2007;27(5):1371–1388

Low VH, Levine MS, Rubesin SE, Laufer I, Herlinger H. Diagnosis of gastric carcinoma: sensitivity of double-contrast barium studies. AJR Am J Roentgenol 1994;162(2):329–334

## Case 5

Rosenberg HK, Serota FT, Koch P, Borden S IV, August CS. Radiographic features of gastrointestinal graft-vs.-host disease. Radiology 1981;138(2):371–374

## Case 6

Choi D, Park H, Lee YR, et al. The most useful findings for diagnosing acute appendicitis on contrast-enhanced helical CT. Acta Radiol 2003;44(6):574–582

Levine CD, Aizenstein O, Lehavi O, Blachar A. Why we miss the diagnosis of appendicitis on abdominal CT: evaluation of imaging features of appendicitis incorrectly diagnosed on CT. AJR Am J Roentgenol 2005;184(3):855–859

## Case 7

Levine MS, Rubesin SE, Laufer I. Pattern approach for diseases of mesenteric small bowel on barium studies. Radiology 2008;249(2):445–460

## Case 8

Singh AK, Gervais DA, Hahn PF, Sagar P, Mueller PR, Novelline RA. Acute epiploic appendagitis and its mimics. Radiographics 2005;25(6):1521–1534

## Case 9

Siegelman ES, Rosen MA. Imaging of hepatic steatosis. Semin Liver Dis 2001;21(1):71–80

## Case 10

Brancatelli G, Baron RL, Peterson MS, Marsh W. Helical CT screening for hepatocellular carcinoma in patients with cirrhosis: frequency and causes of false-positive interpretation. AJR Am J Roentgenol 2003;180(4):1007–1014

## Case 11

Greenberg HM, Goldberg HI, Axel L. Colonic "urticaria" pattern due to early ischemia. Gastrointest Radiol 1981;6(2):145–149

## Case 12

Horton KM, Lawler LP, Fishman EK. CT findings in sclerosing mesenteritis (panniculitis): spectrum of disease. Radiographics 2003;23(6):1561–1567

## Case 13

Görg C, Weide R, Schwerk WB, Köppler H, Havemann K. Ultrasound evaluation of hepatic and splenic microabscesses in the immunocompromised patient: sonographic patterns, differential diagnosis, and follow-up. J Clin Ultrasound 1994;22(9):525–529

## Case 14

Buck JL, Harned RK, Lichtenstein JE, Sobin LH. Peutz-Jeghers syndrome. Radiographics 1992;12(2):365–378

## Case 15

Boscak AR, Al-Hawary M, Ramsburgh SR. Best cases from the AFIP: Adenomyomatosis of the gallbladder. Radiographics 2006;26(3):941–946

## Case 16

Luedtke P, Levine MS, Rubesin SE, Weinstein DS, Laufer I. Radiologic diagnosis of benign esophageal strictures: a pattern approach. Radiographics 2003;23(4):897–909

## Case 17

Levy AD, Murakata LA, Rohrmann CA Jr. Gallbladder carcinoma: radiologic-pathologic correlation. Radiographics 2001;21(2):295–314, 549–555

## Case 18

Levy AD, Remotti HE, Thompson WM, Sobin LH, Miettinen M. Gastrointestinal stromal tumors: radiologic features with pathologic correlation. Radiographics 2003;23(2):283–304, 456, quiz 532

## Case 19

Prasad SR, Wang H, Rosas H, et al. Fat-containing lesions of the liver: radiologic-pathologic correlation. Radiographics 2005;25(2):321–331

## Case 20

Pickhardt PJ. The "hide-bound" bowel sign. Radiology 1999;213(3):837–838

## Case 21

Urrutia M, Mergo PJ, Ros LH, Torres GM, Ros PR. Cystic masses of the spleen: radiologic-pathologic correlation. Radiographics 1996;16(1):107–129

## Case 22

Low VH, Levine MS, Rubesin SE, Laufer I, Herlinger H. Diagnosis of gastric carcinoma: sensitivity of double-contrast barium studies. AJR Am J Roentgenol 1994;162(2):329–334

## Case 23

Klempnauer J, Grothues F, Bektas H, Wahlers T. Acute mesenteric ischemia following cardiac surgery. J Cardiovasc Surg (Torino) 1997;38(6):639–643

Rhee RY, Gloviczki P. Mesenteric venous thrombosis. Surg Clin North Am 1997;77(2):327–338

## Case 24

Kawamoto S, Horton KM, Fishman EK. Pseudomembranous colitis: spectrum of imaging findings with clinical and pathologic correlation. Radiographics 1999;19(4):887–897

Thoeni RF, Cello JP. CT imaging of colitis. Radiology 2006;240(3):623–638

## Case 25

El-Amin LC, Levine MS, Rubesin SE, Shah JN, Kochman ML, Laufer IL. Ileocecal valve: spectrum of normal findings at double-contrast barium enema examination. Radiology 2003;227(1):52–58

Schnur MJ, Seaman WB. Prolapsing neoplasms of the terminal ileum simulating enlarged ileocecal valves. AJR Am J Roentgenol 1980;134(6):1133–1136

## Case 26

Giovagnoni A, Giorgi C, Goteri G. Tumours of the spleen. Cancer Imaging 2005;5(1):73–77

## Case 27

Hiltunen KM, Syrjä H, Matikainen M. Colonic volvulus. Diagnosis and results of treatment in 82 patients. Eur J Surg 1992;158(11-12):607–611

## Case 28

Delis N, Franczak A, Nicolas V, Heyer CM. Incarcerated spigelian hernia mimicking diverticulitis: detection by multidetector computed tomography. Int J Colorectal Dis 2006;21(8):851–853

Miller R, Lifschitz O, Mavor E. Incarcerated Spigelian hernia mimicking obstructing colon carcinoma. Hernia 2008;12(1):87–89

## Case 29

Yee J, Wall SD. Infectious esophagitis. Radiol Clin North Am 1994;32(6):1135–1145

## Case 30

Freeman ME, Rose JL, Forsmark CE, Vauthey JN. Mirizzi syndrome: A rare cause of obstructive jaundice. Dig Dis 1999;17(1):44–48

## Case 31

Kim YH, Blake MA, Harisinghani MG, et al. Adult intestinal intussusception: CT appearances and identification of a causative lead point. Radiographics 2006;26(3):733–744

Sofia S, Casali A, Bolondi L. Sonographic diagnosis of adult intussusception. Abdom Imaging 2001;26(5):483–486

## Case 32

Rubesin SE, Levine MS. Killian-Jamieson diverticula: radiographic findings in 16 patients. AJR Am J Roentgenol 2001;177(1):85–89

## Case 33

Levy AD, Remotti HE, Thompson WM, Sobin LH, Miettinen M. Gastrointestinal stromal tumors: radiologic features with pathologic correlation. Radiographics 2003;23(2):283–304, 456, quiz 532

Sheth S, Horton KM, Garland MR, Fishman EK. Mesenteric neoplasms: CT appearances of primary and secondary tumors and differential diagnosis. Radiographics 2003;23(2):457–473, quiz 535–536

## Case 34

Miller PA, Mezwa DG, Feczko PJ, Jafri ZH, Madrazo BL. Imaging of abdominal hernias. Radiographics 1995;15(2):333–347

## Case 35

Simmons JD. Solitary or multiple nodular lesions in the gastrointestinal tract with central ulceration (bull's-eye or target lesion). Semin Roentgenol 1980;15(4 Pt 2):267–268

## Case 36

Rao PM, Rhea JT, Novelline RA. CT diagnosis of mesenteric adenitis. Radiology 1997;202(1):145–149

## Case 37

Lindberg CG, Hammarström LE, Holmin T, Lundstedt C. Cholangiographic appearance of bile-duct cysts. Abdom Imaging 1998;23(6):611–615

## Case 38

Rao PM. CT of diverticulitis and alternative conditions. Semin Ultrasound CT MR 1999;20(2):86–93

## Case 39

Levy AD, Hobbs CM. From the archives of the AFIP. Meckel diverticulum: radiologic features with pathologic Correlation. Radiographics 2004;24(2):565–587

## Case 40

Kim SJ, Lee JM, Han JK, Kim KH, Lee JY, Choi BI. Peripheral mass-forming cholangiocarcinoma in cirrhotic liver. AJR Am J Roentgenol 2007;189(6):1428–1434

## Case 41

Scotiniotis I, Rubesin SE, Ginsberg GG. Imaging modalities in inflammatory bowel disease. Gastroenterol Clin North Am 1999;28(2):391–421, ix

## Case 42

Levy AD, Rohrmann CA Jr, Murakata LA, Lonergan GJ. Caroli's disease: radiologic spectrum with pathologic correlation. AJR Am J Roentgenol 2002;179(4):1053–1057

## Case 43

Hiltunen KM, Syrjä H, Matikainen M. Colonic volvulus. Diagnosis and results of treatment in 82 patients. Eur J Surg 1992;158(11-12):607–611

## Case 44

Pickhardt PJ, Bhalla S. Primary neoplasms of peritoneal and sub-peritoneal origin: CT findings. Radiographics 2005;25(4):983–995

## Case 45

Iuchtman M, Steiner T, Faierman T, Breitgand A, Bartal G. Post-traumatic intramural duodenal hematoma in children. Isr Med Assoc J 2006;8(2):95–97

## Case 46

Vitellas KM, Keogan MT, Freed KS, et al. Radiologic manifestations of sclerosing cholangitis with emphasis on MR cholangiopancreatography. Radiographics 2000;20(4):959–975, quiz 1108–1109, 1112

## Case 47

Blakeborough A, Chapman AH, Swift S, Culpan G, Wilson D, Sheridan MB. Strictures of the sigmoid colon: barium enema evaluation. Radiology 2001;220(2):343–348

## Case 48

Kawamoto S, Horton KM, Fishman EK. Pseudomembranous colitis: spectrum of imaging findings with clinical and pathologic correlation. Radiographics 1999;19(4):887–897

Ros PR, Buetow PC, Pantograg-Brown L, Forsmark CE, Sobin LH. Pseudomembranous colitis. Radiology 1996;198(1):1–9

Thoeni RF, Cello JP. CT imaging of colitis. Radiology 2006;240(3):623–638

## Case 49

Pickhardt PJ, Levy AD, Rohrmann CA Jr, Abbondanzo SL, Kende AI. Non-Hodgkin's lymphoma of the appendix: clinical and CT findings with pathologic correlation. AJR Am J Roentgenol 2002;178(5):1123–1127

Rubesin SE, Gilchrist AM, Bronner M, et al. Non-Hodgkin lymphoma of the small intestine. Radiographics 1990;10(6):985–998

## Case 50

Blasbalg R, Baroni RH, Costa DN, Machado MCC. MRI features of groove pancreatitis. AJR Am J Roentgenol 2007;189(1):73–80

## Case 51

El-Amin LC, Levine MS, Rubesin SE, Shah JN, Kochman ML, Laufer IL. Ileocecal valve: spectrum of normal findings at double-contrast barium enema examination. Radiology 2003;227(1):52–58

Schnur MJ, Seaman WB. Prolapsing neoplasms of the terminal ileum simulating enlarged ileocecal valves. AJR Am J Roentgenol 1980;134(6):1133–1136

## Case 52

Wittenberg J, Harisinghani MG, Jhaveri K, Varghese J, Mueller PR. Algorithmic approach to CT diagnosis of the abnormal bowel wall. Radiographics 2002;22(5):1093–1107, discussion 1107–1109

## Case 53

Ramachandran I, Sinha R, Rajesh A, Verma R, Maglinte DDT. Multidetector row CT of small bowel tumours. Clin Radiol 2007;62(7):607–614

## Case 54

Rha SE, Ha HK, Lee SH, et al. CT and MR imaging findings of bowel ischemia from various primary causes. Radiographics 2000;20(1):29–42

## Case 55

Buetow PC, Miller DL, Parrino TV, Buck JL. Islet cell tumors of the pancreas: clinical, radiologic, and pathologic correlation in diagnosis and localization. Radiographics 1997;17(2):453–472, quiz 472A–472B

Doppman JL, Miller DL, Chang R, et al. Gastrinomas: localization by means of selective intraarterial injection of secretin. Radiology 1990;174(1):25–29

## Case 56

Kidd R, Freeny PC. Radiographic manifestations of extrinsic processes involving the bowel. Gastrointest Radiol 1982;7(1):21–28

## Case 57

Ho LM, Paulson EK, Thompson WM. Pneumatosis intestinalis in the adult: benign to life-threatening causes. AJR Am J Roentgenol 2007;188(6):1604–1613

Pickhardt PJ. The "hide-bound" bowel sign. Radiology 1999;213(3):837–838

## Case 58

Hirao K, Kikawada M, Hanyu H, Iwamoto T. Sigmoid volvulus showing "a whirl sign" on CT. Intern Med 2006;45(5):331–332

Matsumoto S, Mori H, Okino Y, Tomonari K, Yamada Y, Kiyosue H. Computed tomographic imaging of abdominal volvulus: pictorial essay. Can Assoc Radiol J 2004;55(5):297–303

## Case 59

Harned RK, Buck JL, Sobin LH. The hamartomatous polyposis syndromes: clinical and radiologic features. AJR Am J Roentgenol 1995;164(3):565–571

## Case 60

Buck JL, Hayes WS. From the Archives of the AFIP. Microcystic adenoma of the pancreas. Radiographics 1990;10(2):313–322

## Case 61

Iyomasa S, Kato H, Tachimori Y, Watanabe H, Yamaguchi H, Itabashi M. Carcinosarcoma of the esophagus: a twenty-case study. Jpn J Clin Oncol 1990;20(1):99–106

## Case 62

Kim YH, Saini S, Sahani D, Hahn PF, Mueller PR, Auh YH. Imaging diagnosis of cystic pancreatic lesions: pseudocyst versus nonpseudocyst. Radiographics 2005;25(3):671–685

## Case 63

Rubesin SE, Gilchrist AM, Bronner M, et al. Non-Hodgkin lymphoma of the small intestine. Radiographics 1990;10(6):985–998

## Case 64

Styles RA, Gibb SP, Tarshis A, Silverman ML, Scholz FJ. Esophagogastric polyps: radiographic and endoscopic findings. Radiology 1985;154(2):307–311

## Case 65

Kaufman LB, Yeh BM, Breiman RS, Joe BN, Qayyum A, Coakley FV. Inferior vena cava filling defects on CT and MRI. AJR Am J Roentgenol 2005;185(3):717–726

## Case 66

Cronin CG, Lohan DG, Blake MA, Roche C, McCarthy P, Murphy JM. Retroperitoneal fibrosis: a review of clinical features and imaging findings. AJR Am J Roentgenol 2008;191(2):423–431

## Case 67

Luedtke P, Levine MS, Rubesin SE, Weinstein DS, Laufer I. Radiologic diagnosis of benign esophageal strictures: a pattern approach. Radiographics 2003;23(4):897–909

## Case 68

Grayson DE, Abbott RM, Levy AD, Sherman PM. Emphysematous infections of the abdomen and pelvis: a pictorial review. Radiographics 2002;22(3):543–561

## Case 69

Thoeni RF, Goldberg HI, Ominsky S, Cello JP. Detection of gastritis by single- and double-contrast radiography. Radiology 1983; 148(3):621–626

## Case 70

Hussain SM, Terkivatan T, Zondervan PE, et al. Focal nodular hyperplasia: findings at state-of-the-art MR imaging, US, CT, and pathologic analysis. Radiographics 2004;24(1):3–17, discussion 18–19

## Case 71

Young MA, Rose S, Reynolds JC. Gastrointestinal manifestations of scleroderma. Rheum Dis Clin North Am 1996;22(4):797–823

## Case 72

Menon KV, Shah V, Kamath PS. The Budd-Chiari syndrome. N Engl J Med 2004;350(6):578–585

## Case 73

Gore RM, Berlin JW, Mehta UK, Newmark GM, Yaghmai V. GI carcinoid tumours: appearance of the primary and detecting metastases. Best Pract Res Clin Endocrinol Metab 2005;19(2):245–263

## Case 74

Wittenberg J, Harisinghani MG, Jhaveri K, Varghese J, Mueller PR. Algorithmic approach to CT diagnosis of the abnormal bowel wall. Radiographics 2002;22(5):1093–1107, discussion 1107–1109

## Case 75

Heithold DL, Tucker JG, Lucas GW. Appendiceal intussusception as a manifestation of mucinous cystadenoma of the appendix: an interesting clinical entity. Am Surg 1997;63(5):390–391

Kim SH, Lim HK, Lee WJ, Lim JH, Byun JY. Mucocele of the appendix: ultrasonographic and CT findings. Abdom Imaging 1998;23(3): 292–296

## Case 76

Fry RD, Kodner IJ. Rectovaginal fistula. Surg Annu 1995;27:113–131

## Case 77

McDermott VG, Low VH, Keogan MT, Lawrence JA, Paulson EK. Malignant melanoma metastatic to the gastrointestinal tract. AJR Am J Roentgenol 1996;166(4):809–813

## Case 78

Gold CH, Morley JE, Viljoen M, Tim LO, de Fomseca M, Kalk WJ. Gastric acid secretion and serum gastrin levels in patients with chronic renal failure on regular hemodialysis. Nephron 1980;25(2):92–95

Rubesin SE, Levine MS, Laufer I. Double-contrast upper gastrointestinal radiography: a pattern approach for diseases of the stomach. Radiology 2008;246(1):33–48

## Case 79

Ichikawa T, Federle MP, Grazioli L, Madariaga J, Nalesnik M, Marsh W. Fibrolamellar hepatocellular carcinoma: imaging and pathologic findings in 31 recent cases. Radiology 1999;213(2):352–361

## Case 80

Ott DJ. Radiographic techniques and efficacy in evaluating esophageal dysphagia. Dysphagia 1990;5(4):192–203

## Case 81

Buetow PC, Buck JL, Pantongrag-Brown L, et al. Biliary cystadenoma and cystadenocarcinoma: clinical-imaging-pathologic correlations with emphasis on the importance of ovarian stroma. Radiology 1995;196(3):805–810

## Case 82

Carucci LR, Levine MS, Rubesin SE, Laufer I. Upper gastrointestinal tract barium examination of postbulbar duodenal ulcers. AJR Am J Roentgenol 2004;182(4):927–930

## Case 83

Kawamoto S, Soyer PA, Fishman EK, Bluemke DA. Nonneoplastic liver disease: evaluation with CT and MR imaging. Radiographics 1998;18(4):827–848

## Case 84

Rubesin SE, Saul SH, Laufer I, Levine MS. Carpet lesions of the colon. Radiographics 1985;5:537–552

## Case 85

Takayassu TC, Marchiori E, Eiras A, et al. Telangiectatic adenoma - computed tomography and magnetic resonance findings: a case report and review of the literature. Cases J 2009;2(1):24

## Case 86

Takeyama N, Gokan T, Ohgiya Y, et al. CT of internal hernias. Radiographics 2005;25(4):997–1015

## Case 87

Wittenberg J, Harisinghani MG, Jhaveri K, Varghese J, Mueller PR. Algorithmic approach to CT diagnosis of the abnormal bowel wall. Radiographics 2002;22(5):1093–1107, discussion 1107–1109

## Case 88

Horton KM, Abrams RA, Fishman EK. Spiral CT of colon cancer: imaging features and role in management. Radiographics 2000; 20(2):419–430

## Case 89

Meyer JE. Radiography of the distal colon and rectum after irradiation of carcinoma of the cervix. AJR Am J Roentgenol 1981;136(4):691–699

## Case 90

Lepanto L, Arzoumanian Y, Gianfelice D, et al. Helical CT with CT angiography in assessing periampullary neoplasms: identification of vascular invasion. Radiology 2002;222(2):347–352

## Case 91

Menuck L. Plain film findings of gastric volvulus herniating into the chest. AJR Am J Roentgenol 1976;126(6):1169–1174

## Case 92

Pickhardt PJ, Levy AD, Rohrmann CA Jr, Kende AI. Primary neoplasms of the appendix: radiologic spectrum of disease with pathologic correlation. Radiographics 2003;23(3):645–662

## Case 93

Matsumoto S, Mori H, Okino Y, Tomonari K, Yamada Y, Kiyosue H. Computed tomographic imaging of abdominal volvulus: pictorial essay. Can Assoc Radiol J 2004;55(5):297–303

## Case 94

Ott DJ. Radiographic techniques and efficacy in evaluating esophageal dysphagia. Dysphagia 1990;5(4):192–203

## Case 95

Kalra MK, Maher MM, Mueller PR, Saini S. State-of-the-art imaging of pancreatic neoplasms. Br J Radiol 2003;76(912):857–865

## Case 96

Low VH, Levine MS, Rubesin SE, Laufer I, Herlinger H. Diagnosis of gastric carcinoma: sensitivity of double-contrast barium studies. AJR Am J Roentgenol 1994;162(2):329–334

Shindoh N, Nakagawa T, Ozaki Y, Kyogoku S, Sumi Y, Katayama H. Overlooked gastric carcinoma: pitfalls in upper gastrointestinal radiology. Radiology 2000;217(2):409–414

## Case 97

Prasad SR, Wang H, Rosas H, et al. Fat-containing lesions of the liver: radiologic-pathologic correlation. Radiographics 2005;25(2):321–331

## Case 98

Sulkin TVC, O'Neill H, Amin AI, Moran B. CT in pseudomyxoma peritonei: a review of 17 cases. Clin Radiol 2002;57(7):608–613

## Case 99

Yagan N, Auh YH, Fisher A. Extension of air into the right perirenal space after duodenal perforation: CT findings. Radiology 2009;250(3):740–748

## Case 100

Cole TJ, Turner MA. Manifestations of gastrointestinal disease on chest radiographs. Radiographics 1993;13(5):1013–1034

# Index

Note: Locators refer to case number. Locators in **boldface** indicate primary diagnosis.